My Race with Prostate Cancer

My Race with Prostate Cancer

◆

A Runner's Journal

Allan P. Drew

iUniverse, Inc.
New York Lincoln Shanghai

My Race with Prostate Cancer
A Runner's Journal

iUniverse books may be ordered through booksellers or by contacting:

iUniverse
2021 Pine Lake Road, Suite 100
Lincoln, NE 68512
www.iuniverse.com
1-800-Authors (1-800-288-4677)

Because of the dynamic nature of the Internet, any Web addresses or links contained in this book may have changed since publication and may no longer be valid.

The information, ideas, and suggestions in this book are not intended as a substitute for professional medical advice. Before following any suggestions contained in this book, you should consult your personal physician. Neither the author nor the publisher shall be liable or responsible for any loss or damage allegedly arising as a consequence of your use or application of any information or suggestions in this book.

ISBN: 978-0-595-45830-1 (pbk)
ISBN: 978-0-595-90130-2 (ebk)

Printed in the United States of America

This book is dedicated to all masters athletes who, by their choice of a physically active lifestyle, improve their own level of health and fitness and so provide inspiration to others who may choose to begin an exercise program or remain competitive in their sport as they grow older.

Contents

1

Introduction

I approached my annual physical in May of 1996 like any other. I expected it to be short and sweet, merely a formality, as I had enjoyed excellent health all my life and, as a runner, was in top physical shape. I had no indications that anything between my ears and toes was amiss in any way, nor less than fully functional. I had always gone for an annual physical stemming from the habit that began as a child. There were probably a few years in between high school and my early thirties, when I entered the professional job market as an academician, when I was not regular in my health checkups. Then, they were taken out of necessity for Peace Corps entry purposes, for college admissions or when there had been a specific problem to deal with. Outside of that, and especially after my marriage at age 39, the physicals had been regular and almost without exception from a medical doctor's point of view, unproductive and uninteresting. There was never much of anything wrong with me that would pique my family doctor's interest, ease his professional boredom, or cause him to pull the medical encyclopedia down from the shelf to look up something he had rarely encountered before. In short, I had been lulled into a sense of complacency in regard to my annual physicals. At age 53, I expected my visit to the doctor to show nothing out of the ordinary and thought it to be unproductive time that could be better spent at my academic obligations as a forest physiological ecologist. I went to the doctor out of habit. I would get it over with, then get back to the office and not think about it for another year.

For the past 14 years I had been a "runner," as distinct from a "jogger." I was one who trained for competition and ran in road races as well as doing sprints and field events as a masters track athlete. I belonged to the

1

Syracuse Chargers Track Club and regularly participated in sanctioned events. I was a volunteer at events as well and served on the Board of Directors. Running was, and still is, an important part of my life. I enjoy it for the challenge it presents—the training for personal fitness, the competition with fellow athletes, and the ultimate challenge which is to improve upon one's own performance, to challenge one's self to achieve something that is mentally and physically difficult.

The term, "masters," when applied to running, generally refers to a runner aged 40 or above, someone who participates in competitive running beyond an age when many are more actively engaged in careers, raising a family or have long since decided to leave their sport. Masters runners are often athletes who had successful careers in college or even Olympians who find they retain a love of running and competition even though many of their peers have long ago hung up their track shoes. Eamon Coghlin, former Irish Olympian, who is one of the few milers to run a sub 3:50 mile indoors, having run a 3:48.78 in 1983, broke the 4-minute barrier with a 3:58.15 in 1994 in Boston at age 41. As such, he was the first masters runner over 40 to run a sub-4 minute mile.

Some masters runners, however, are individuals who have come to the sport late in life perhaps as a way to lose weight or to join their offspring who are runners, and have discovered a latent ability or love of running that has stuck with them. Not all masters runners are like Eamon Coghlin; the vast majority are not. Most, in fact, are people who were never great athletes, but found something in running that made their lives better, healthier, that gave them a feeling of accomplishment.

Like the annual physicals, running was something I had done since childhood, and it has taught me discipline, among other qualities. To reach peak performances requires regular training. Whether one feels like running or not on any given day is somewhat beside the point. Training requires adherence to a schedule in order to achieve maximum cardiovascular efficiency and muscular strength that translate into faster times on the track or roads. Discipline is learned, and it extends to other areas of life. Once a runner realizes that he or she has made personal improvements in the sport, and that such improvement is repeatable, once the proper techniques are learned, it is a natural extension to be disciplined in other areas of life such as in the workplace, academic study or even in such singular tasks as learning to drive an automobile or losing weight.

2

Coach Newton

My running career began with track and cross-country at York High School in Elmhurst, Illinois between 1957–61 where I had the good fortune to be coached by Joe Newton, one of the great motivational coaches in the sport. Coach Newton's cross-country teams have won 26 state titles in 47 years of coaching at York, and in 2004 won a national championship at the Nike Team Nationals. He has been named Illinois High School Coach of the Year once in track and 15 times in cross-country. In addition, Joe Newton has the distinction of being the first high school coach ever selected to be a U.S. Olympic coach when he served as an assistant manager in track and field at the 1988 Olympic Games held in Seoul, South Korea. In 1998, he was inducted into the U.S. Track Coaches Hall of Fame.

Coach Newton's inspirational teaching was a dominant force throughout my early years and into adult life. He taught us athletes the benefits of hard work, discipline and commitment. Joe Newton's philosophy is more than a philosophy of how to be a good runner. It is a philosophy of life—of how to be a successful person. In his words, "Too often we get distracted by what is outside our control. You can't do anything about **YESTERDAY**. The door to the past has been shut, you can do nothing about **TOMORROW**. It is yet to come. However, tomorrow is in large part determined by what you do today. So make today a **MASTERPIECE**. You have control over that." Or, this. "I have discovered a rule more important in life than running. You have to apply yourself each day to become a little better. By applying yourself to the task of becoming a little better each and every day, over a period of time, you will become **A LOT** better, only then will you be able to approach being the best you can be. It begins by trying to make each day count and knowing you can **NEVER** make up for a lost day."

Following high school, although I did not participate in intercollegiate track, I did participate informally in other sports such as swimming, handball, skiing and baseball throughout ten years of college. I did not become active again as a pure runner until my late thirties when I moved to Syracuse, New York where I joined the faculty of the State University of New York's College of Environmental Science and Forestry. At this time, I discovered and joined the Syracuse Chargers, an organization that successfully reawakened a dormant love and enthusiasm for running. In masters track and field I rediscovered my roots as a high school athlete.

The Syracuse Chargers Track Club is one of the premier running clubs in the Northeast if not the country. They are dedicated to the development of all aspects of Athletics in Central New York, including support for youth development programs and the encouragement of individuals of all ages and abilities to participate in local, regional, national and international track & field, long distance and race walking events. Under the able direction of Nate and Evelyn White, Dave Oja and others, the Chargers Track Club has grown into a large organization offering quality programs for its many members. The Chargers facilitated my development as a competitive runner through my 40's and 50's. Participation in indoor and outdoor track meets and road races, leading the Chargers youth program, volunteering at events, and serving on its Board, all fostered the development of a renewed interest in track and field as a sport. The Chargers Track Club, through the camaraderie of other masters runners, their dedication, commitment and love of the sport, has become the second major motivational force next to Coach Joe Newton years earlier, to direct and focus a major part of my life around running.

3

Physical Exam, Biopsy and a Dire Prognosis

All went well at the doctor's at first. My blood pressure was a robust 110/66 with a resting pulse of 62. My heart and lungs checked out fine. There was no sign of hernia and my knee jerked appropriately when Dr. Peter Grendle hit it with the rubber hammer. We were about finished when I remembered the Time magazine article of April, 1995, I had recently read about Norman Schwartzkopf and his battle with prostate cancer. I had learned of a simple blood test that Schwartzkopf had taken that led to his initial diagnosis. The prostate-specific antigen or PSA test would indicate the state of prostate health. In young men with healthy prostates it should produce a level of PSA of less than 4.0 ng/ml (since revised to less than 2.5 ng/ml). I knew from the Time article and from talking to older men that I was within the age range where prostate disease can become a concern.

Before my physical was over, I asked Dr. Grendle if I might be tested for prostate health with the PSA blood test. He replied, "Well, I don't recommend it as a matter of course because there are false positives and false negatives often associated with the test." He explained that elevated PSA tests don't always indicate prostate cancer and may lead a person into a series of uncomfortable and complex diagnostic tests. Also, up to 20 percent of men with prostate cancer will have a normal PSA level (American Cancer Society, 1999). Additionally, a man's PSA level tends to increase with age, and can mask early cancer that may be present. Nevertheless, I said I would still like to be given the test. Something so simple seemed hardly worth passing by, especially when the statistics I had read about prostate cancer seemed so ominous.

In the U.S., prostate cancer causes almost 30,000 deaths a year with about 220,000 new cases diagnosed annually, making it the second leading cause of mortality among men after lung cancer. A boy born today has a 13 percent chance of developing prostate cancer, and a 3 percent chance of dying from it. The disease hardly ever appears before age 40, but becomes more common with increasing age among older men. Eight out of ten patients are older than 65. For reasons not known, African-Americans are twice as likely to contract the disease as European-Americans.

Dr. Grendle relented and a nurse took the blood sample. In a few days, I received a phone call from the doctor's office that my PSA test reading was 7.3 ng/ml. Dr. Grendle subsequently explained that he was concerned enough by the elevated reading that he wanted me to see a urologist. He had detected some slight swelling on the digital rectal exam, a procedure where a gloved finger is inserted up the rectum and the prostate examined by feel, and had dismissed it, but felt that the above normal PSA reading should be investigated further. My prior physical had also indicated a slight swelling of the prostate, but my doctor felt it to be normal for my age. After age 40, the prostate gland, for unknown reasons, grows larger. This is not harmful unless it exerts pressure on the urethra, making urination difficult.

I thought little of the referral, feeling that probably there was some simple explanation for the elevated PSA. In any case, I reasoned, I had had none of the symptoms of prostate disease such as swelling of the gland leading to difficulties or pain with urination. My first visit to the urologist, Dr. Walter Stonehouse, led to a second one. His initial reaction was that he wanted to check me out further with ultrasound and possibly a tissue biopsy, and gave me pamphlets to read on the biopsy procedure. On June 21st, I went in for the biopsy.

During the procedure, while lying on my side, a small tissue sampling needle contained in a probe was shot into my prostate from inside the rectum while the doctor observed the organ on an ultrasound screen. The sampling needle was sent into areas of the prostate that the doctor deemed suspicious. When the probe containing the needle was withdrawn it contained a small bit of prostate tissue that was then sent to a medical lab for analysis. I felt a dull pain when the needle went in as it did 8 times, 4 on each side of the prostate. I was cautioned that I might notice blood in my urine for a few days or in semen for several weeks. The biopsy wounds eventually heal. I walked away from the medical office feeling some slight pain, but otherwise with no ill effects.

The prostate gland wraps around the urethra, the tube that carries urine from the bladder. Its main function is to produce semen, the fluid that carries sperm out of the body. Symptoms appear if swelling of the prostate presses on the urethra, causing urine to pool and stagnate in the bladder and infection to occur (prostatitis). If cancer is present, it may again produce swelling and pressure on the urethra. Or, as in older men, the prostate may swell and restrict the flow of urine, resulting in a thin stream and/ or incompletely emptied bladder. In the latter case, the bladder walls thicken to hold the backed-up urine, producing a constant feeling of needing to empty the bladder. Such problems associated with an enlarged prostate are common in older men, even though cancer may not be present. Many men older than 50 suffer from BPH, or benign prostatic hyperplasia, a non-cancerous enlargement of the prostate gland. BPH is a problem for about 25 percent of men in their 50's and for half of men over 75.

My biopsy was on Friday. The following Wednesday I had the result. I was home in the morning when the phone rang. A nurse calling from the urologist's office announced, "Mr. Drew, I have your biopsy results. You've tested positive for cancer." There was no suggestion that I meet in person with my urologist or even that I assume a comfortable position before receiving the test results. It was a clear, unadulterated statement of the biopsy analysis. The nurse said it in a cheerful matter-of-fact tone as though she were remarking on the likelihood of the sun rising the following morning. Its impact on me was anything but cheerful. I felt my heart beat faster at her words and an incipient despondency closed in. She went on—"We've arranged for you to have a bone scan tomorrow morning at Crouse-Irving Hospital." The complete body scan would tell my urologist if the cancer had spread beyond the prostate to my bones. This would be the worst possible scenario. The best I could hope for was that nothing would show up on the bone scan. Knowing now that I had cancer, it was essential to determine if the cancer had spread beyond the prostate. Treatment would be based on the stage of development of the cancer and where it was located in my body.

I have since considered the manner in which I was definitively informed that I had cancer. From the standpoint of the physician's office staff, a simple phone call from a nurse is the easiest, most expedient way of dispensing a test result. When the result is life threatening, however, I am not sure but what something of a more personal approach should be employed. From the patient's perspective, a visit to the doctor might be more effective. In my case, it would have allowed me to discuss the test result with someone better able than I to understand its true significance. Secondly, it would have given me the opportunity to talk man-to-man with someone more familiar to me than a nurse I had never met. Finally, when the phone rings, it is always a surprise—lives are never planned to accommodate phone calls. They always interrupt something. Luckily, I was at home. I could just as easily have been in the middle of a committee meeting at work or in the midst of discussions with a potential graduate student. In my case, I was at home alone. I would have preferred to have been with my wife or doctor when receiving such news. On the other hand, I can understand how some men, if asked to come in to their doctor's office to receive their test results, would conjure up all sorts of negative scenarios, causing needless worry and anxiety. Maybe it is best to get it done and over with by a simple phone call rather then keeping the patient in suspense any longer than is necessary. I expect that most doctors think of such things when considering how best to bring bad news to a patient.

I asked a doctor friend how he relates bad health news to his patients. He replied that he tries to be with the person when he has something very negative to discuss and to have a plan in mind for what to do next. Many doctors, like my urologist, are probably just too busy to meet with each person individually.

4

Handling Fear

On the day I learned of my cancer, I had agreed to take my 11-year-old daughter, Katie, and her visiting friend from Tucson, Irene, along with my 8-year-old son, Will, to the Burnet Park Zoo for the afternoon. In my state of shock over the test results, it was a forced effort to accompany my kids and Irene around the Zoo for 3 hours. None of them knew what I knew—that their father was now the owner of a potentially deadly disease. I had not tried to reach my wife, Beth. She had clearly stated that she wanted to be present with me when told the biopsy results. She did not want to receive them at work over the telephone. Perhaps the animals at the Zoo would provide some distraction for the mixture of feelings I now possessed—fear, anxiety over the bone scan, uncertainty over the future—and of which none had been present only hours before.

The prior Tuesday I had run a fast 200 meter race in a local track meet, 27.3 seconds, which for me at age 53 was better than I had run in several years. As I had run "the 200" for a number of years, even as a high school track athlete, I knew what I could do and where my peak performance lay. I had trained well this summer, adopted some new training methods and set several P.R.'s (personal records), so was feeling confident in my body's ability to respond physically to the demands of training and to the ultimate test of competition. Two-and-a-half weeks earlier I had won the Empire State Senior Games 400 meters in 62.5 seconds in the 50–54 age group, a performance that eventually placed me at 62nd in the nation according to the U.S. Masters Track and Field ratings. I was feeling good, running well, and looking forward to the rest of the summer. Twenty-four hours later I would reach a depth of despair and anxiety that was at least the equal, but opposite, of my recent feelings of mental exhilaration and psychological well being over my running accomplishments.

The Zoo trip was not pleasant, the animals were not the diversion I had hoped they would be, and an afternoon with my kids and their friend, normally a fun time, was anything but that. Yet, I was glad that I had gone to the Zoo on that day because it was something I had planned to do and had looked forward to. As difficult as the trip was, it was important to me that my newly discovered disease not be allowed to derail my carefully laid plans for that day. Although my prostate was presently less than healthy, the cancer need not be allowed to spread to infect and destroy other areas of life. Had I chosen to cancel the Zoo trip, nothing would have been gained. The cancer would still have been there, the bone scan still upcoming on the 'morrow, and Beth would still need to know the results of my biopsy when she returned from work at five o'clock. Canceling the Zoo excursion would only have cost my kids and their friend a nice afternoon and allowed me to more fully engage the destructive tendencies of my mind as I wallowed at home in distress. Perhaps I still gave vent to some of those tendencies while at the Zoo, but at least others did not have to suffer because of my disease, and I later felt somewhat pleased with myself that I had been able to carry on with plans in spite of being in an anxiety-ridden, emotionally distraught state of mind. Social discourse and exchange of pleasantries were conducted with difficulty at best, not with their usual spontaneity, but I had at least taken an important first step in confronting and dealing with my disease. I was seeing the necessity for dealing with it as one of many facets of my whole life and not as a separate overriding entity. The rest of my life, exclusive of the cancer, could be kept reasonably healthy and well if I gave it that kind of attention. Or, it could be allowed to fester and deteriorate as I focused completely on the prostate condition. This attitude would be exemplified many more times during the months ahead and was to become a source of inner sustenance to me in dealing with my own emotions and feelings about my cancer.

5

The Urologist Explains

Dr. Stonehouse had scheduled a Tuesday appointment to discuss with Beth and me the results of the bone scan I had taken the previous Thursday morning, as well as details of the biopsy. The actual scan procedure was a simple one. I was given a tecnitium-99 tracer orally, then told to come back in two hours for the scan after the tracer had worked its way throughout my system. I recall looking around the waiting room at others and wondering if they were there for any reasons similar to my own and if so, how they must be as adept as I imagined I was in hiding one's true feelings. None seemed to be particularly upset or ill at ease. I still had no idea whether my cancer was contained within my prostate or if it had spread beyond. In such circumstances, it is easy for the mind to conjure up scenarios that are at odds with reality. Fears became magnified out of proportion as my anxieties grew and what the bone scan might show became like a lump in the back of my mind that would not go away. I have come to realize that what one knows to be true is often not nearly as terrifying as the uncertainty associated with not knowing. The five days of waiting for the bone scan results were fraught with stress. I attempted to carry on with life as usual, but it was a pretense—always there was the obsession with my condition and what I might learn on Tuesday. How would I respond if I learned that the cancer was in my bones? Was I about to become a statistic? One of the three percent? What of all that Beth and I had planned for the rest of our lives? Would I see our kids grow up? These questions passed through my mind as I went through the motions of life. I had not prepared for the worst, but I had great apprehension over what was to come.

Beth and I walked into my urologist's waiting room and I signed in with the secretary behind the desk. I was told to take a seat, that the doctor would meet with me shortly. We seated ourselves in a room where a half dozen other patients were within eyeshot, it not earshot, of a television tuned to a daytime talk show. Some were watching the show; others were reading magazines; several seemed to be just sitting, gazing off into space. The talk show host was interviewing a young woman who had disposed of her newly born child in a dumpster. She was obviously scared as she replied to the host's questions. I wondered how much of her demeanor was related to being on national TV and how much to guilt over what she had done. Then, the host brought on the father of the child and the interviewing continued.

I found myself wishing even more than ever that I was anywhere else but in that waiting room. If my own anxiety was uncomfortable to deal with, listening to the talk show only compounded my uneasy state of mind. Daytime talk shows seem to seek out and exploit the most strange, immoral and obscene sorts of social behaviors in people in order to attract viewers. Not only do they exploit the visiting individuals, but the viewing audience as well since the latter are being attracted to television programming that appeals to the most prurient of interests with little redeeming qualities. In my case, I was being forced to watch something that, frankly, added mental nausea to my already stressed psyche. As some in the waiting room seemed interested in the show and no one emerged to change the television channel, I resolved to lodge a complaint with the office staff over their choice of entertainment. Perhaps no one else in the room was facing a life-threatening illness. But does one have to be in that situation in order to recognize that what their eyes are seeing and ears hearing is pathological? Just then, my name was called.

As Beth and I walked into Dr. Stonehouse's office, I took a final deep breath. I was ready. My doctor's outward countenance revealed nothing of what my test had shown. He offered us chairs in front of his desk and proceeded to discuss prostate cancer in general and methods of treatment. He went on for awhile, then he said casually, "Your bone scan was negative." His words brought a flush of relief to my apprehensive anticipation. Of the four biopsies on the right side of my prostate, two showed cancer; none of the four on the left side had indicated cancer. He went on to explain that prostate cancer is described by its stage—how far the cancer has spread, and its grade—how vigorous and likely are the cancer cells to spread. My stage, according to tables in Patrick Walsh's The Prostate—A Guide for Men and the Women Who Love Them was "T2a" meaning that my cancer was presently palpable, involving less than half of one lobe. It was graded according to the Gleason score (0 to 10) as a 7 which indicated a mildly aggressive rate of cell differentiation and a "significant cancer." The TNM system defines the size of the tumor with a "T" rating being less serious than an "N" or "M" rating. The Gleason score indicates how well defined the cells are with the higher numbers indicating a more amorphous, less defined state and therefore a more serious problem.

Patrick C. Walsh, Professor of Urology and Director of the Brady Urological Institute at The Johns Hopkins Medical Institutions in Baltimore, Maryland, did significant research on surgical procedures with the prostate, pioneering the development of what is termed "the bloodless field." Prior to his work, it had been difficult to see the tissues involved in surgery due to significant blood loss, so accuracy with a scalpel was less than ideal. Walsh also developed methods for saving the neurovascular bundles to either side of the prostate which are involved in penile erections. As a result of his research, impotence following prostate surgery has been reduced and the present-day surgical procedures are more reliable. His 1995 book, and later, his 2001 update (Walsh and Worthington, 2001), written for the layman, is the bible on the prostate. My urologist recommended it and I similarly do so for anyone searching for a readable, authoritative source of information, especially for anyone evaluating alternatives.

Exactly when cancer cells escape the prostate and what causes them to migrate to other parts of the body is not known, but Rafii and Lyden (2005) have shown that bone marrow progenitors prime the organ in which the tumor cells will implant, preparing the organ for cancer cell growth. Men with early stages of cancer can have metastases well before anything is palpable. Yet, more advanced stages than mine have been known where the cancer was confined solely to the prostate. Once the cancer has escaped the prostate, it cannot be cured, only treated, and there is often some reduction in life span. Once it reaches the bones, the average life expectancy is three years. Walsh's book contains a table that used the PSA test score, the clinical stage of the cancer and the Gleason score to predict the probability that the cancer will be completely confined to the prostate. For me, the chances that my cancer had not jumped ship were 51 percent—not good betting odds. Although it was not in my bones, it could still be outside of the prostate infecting nearby lymph nodes or seminal vesicles, for example. Such could only be determined by lymph node examination during surgery. It was facts such as these that, although they helped me to develop a medical understanding of the possible progression of my disease, also brought me face-to-face with my own mortality. In retrospect, I would not have traded ignorance of my condition for understanding. It was knowledge itself that had initially brought me to request the PSA test from my general practitioner. I could live with the facts better than I could the degree of uncertainty that medical illiteracy would bring. I decided it was best to know what was happening in my tissues and organs because then I could assume some responsibility for their health and preservation. In essence, I could make more intelligent decisions regarding my treatment.

6

Spirituality and Stress Release

When confronted with a serious life-threatening illness, most people will use any resources they may have at their own disposal in addition to those their doctor might suggest. Beth and I had early on decided we would approach my illness as a team, sharing in discussions with my urologist and with each other as critical decisions were made. As Christians, we believe in the power of prayer and in the presence of God in our lives as an uplifting, healing force. Our religious faith has been an important part of our individual and married lives and in this case served as an important personal resource. Likewise, our church community was a special resource of supportive, understanding individuals. Their calls, cards and concerns were uplifting. They helped me realize I was not alone in my fight with prostate cancer. I learned of other men who had been treated for prostate cancer and others with severe non-cancerous prostate conditions. Early on, I had decided I would be open with others about my disease. Prostate cancer can have ominous implications for those who contract it. Only by sharing our experiences in open dialogue can men come to understand the disease and its treatment. If my being open with others has influenced just one person to have a regular PSA test, then it will have been successful. I made certain that when my condition was known to me, others knew of it too. I did not attempt to hide anything. Although I never became part of any formal or informal prostate cancer support group, I have always felt that simple openness and honesty with others has great therapeutic value. Local chapters of the American Cancer Society sponsor the "Man to Man" program of education and support for men who have prostate cancer and for their families. At their monthly meetings, there are speakers on various topics related to prostate cancer, there are support groups if those are needed, and there is the opportunity to ask questions of others who may have greater knowledge on the subject through experience or self-learning than one's self.

The power of the human mind can be a great force in healing. Twenty years ago I took a course called Silva Mind Control. Jose Silva, the founder, believed that all people have the innate power to tap their own psychic abilities which they are taught how to do in the basic course. Using an electroencephalograph, Silva developed easily learned methods that have been taught in more than 100 countries, in 29 different languages for more than 30 years. In the Silva course, one is taught how to use the untapped potential of the human mind to achieve healthy goals for oneself and for others. Silva graduates have used basic Mind Control methods to diagnose disease, to heal themselves and friends and to achieve success in business or in their families.

Armed with the knowledge of Silva techniques, three days after learning of my cancer, I began "programming" a healthy outcome to my situation. In the Silva course I was taught how to go to "the alpha level" and once there suggest to myself the positive results I hoped to achieve. At "the alpha level" one reaches a deeper state of mind where brain waves slow to 10 cycles per second and autosuggestions, called "programming," are more likely to be actualized subconsciously than at everyday waking levels of thought. Several times a day I repeated phrases such as these while at "alpha": "Everyday in every way I am becoming healthier, and healthier and healthier." "Positive thoughts bring me benefits and advantages I desire." "I expect the best and with God's help will attain the best." "Unhealthy cells cannot survive in my prostate or anywhere else in my body. They are gradually being replaced by healthy, normal functioning cells."

Another mental technique which helped me during my period of diagnosis, treatment and recovery and which has been a part of my daily routine for over 35 years is transcendental meditation, or TM, as it is popularly known. Twice a day for 20 minutes each time I practice an ancient type of meditation that uses a personally-designed mantra to achieve a more refined, subtler state of thought. In the process, stress is said to be released. My subjective experience over many years is that this is actually what happens during the practice of TM. Stress is eliminated from human bodies in various ways—by sleep, by exercise and gradually during our conscious waking hours of each day. Transcendental meditation achieves stress release in a deliberate way that is rapid and effective. Prostate cancer is not only a stressor of the physical body, but oft accompanying fears and anxieties cause mental and psychological stresses to develop as well. It is therefore necessary to treat the disease as well as the stress that arises out of knowing that one has a potentially serious disease. Meditation, for me, has always been an effective way of handling my daily accumulation of stress.

In addition to TM and Silva Mind Control, I sought relief from the stress associated with knowing I had prostate cancer, but as yet not knowing the extent of it nor what to do about it, through my regular running regime. Since taking up competitive running at age 39, I had worked out on the track or on roads three times a week nearly year round, missing workouts only for sickness or other events beyond my control. A fourth day included a 45 minute weight training program in the gym designed to strengthen all the major muscle groups in the body. At times, such as when I was trying to build rather than maintain strength, I spent part of a second day a week in weight training.

My running workout has always been something I have felt good about after it was over. Non-runners have asked me why it is in my workouts that I appear not to smile, even hold a grimace at times, when in fact I profess to enjoy running. I have to admit that I do not always enjoy running while training. Hard running, the kind it takes to reach one's peak of performance, is hard work. It is not always enjoyable, but the benefits justify the means. The feeling of being in good physical shape is indescribable, especially to a non-athlete. The surge of endorphins and the pleasantly relaxed, but not exhausted, feeling after recovering from a hard workout has always been satisfying. It has been an indication of my being in top condition that has allowed me to continue to compete in my chosen sport at an age when the TV, couch and a beer are the extent of "exercise" for many men.

Mike Tymn, regular columnist for National Masters News, a monthly periodical for runners and track and field athletes over 30, writes how the natural decline in human vitality with age can be slowed through regular exercise. Writing in the May, 1997 issue, Mike relates the work of Walter M. Bortz, II, M.D., a professor of internal medicine at the Stanford University Medical School and former president of the American Geriatrics Society whose research shows that the average sedentary person loses physical vitality at about two-percent a year beginning at age 30 (Bortz, 1996). His results are based on the VO2 max test that measures the efficiency with which we take in oxygen. The physical decline that comes with aging is pretty much linear from 30 to at least 70. Yet, a person who maintains an active lifestyle loses only around one-half of a percent a year. Thus, he or she loses roughly 20 percent between the ages of 30 and 70 rather than 80 percent for a sedentary person. At age 39 I could run 200 meters in 25.8 seconds. At age 53 my time had fallen to 27.3 seconds, a loss of 1.5 seconds in 14 years or a decrease of 0.42 percent per year. Thus, my own experience corroborated Dr. Bortz' research results.

After learning of my positive biopsy results, I continued to train for the Masters Track and Field events in the Empire State Games to be held at the University of Buffalo July 26th. My biopsy result came through exactly a month to the day before I was to compete in what, to me, has always been an extremely challenging, but satisfying competition. In between was a local tune-up meet. I had not anticipated having to give up a pint of my blood, however, in the week before the Games.

7

Sorting Through Medical Options

As Beth and I sat in Dr. Stonehouse's office, my doctor outlined my alternatives. Since my cancer had not spread to my bones, there was a decent chance (51%) that it was contained within the organ. For those such as myself, a surgical operation called a "radical prostatectomy" is a recommended option. Cutting out and removing the entire organ, then rebuilding the urinary system, gets rid of the cancer, but of course also means life without a prostate gland. For some men this operation is not a choice due to feared side effects of sexual impotence and incontinence. These are, however, much less problematic nowadays due to surgical advances such as those developed by Patrick Walsh. Still, anyone undergoing a radical prostatectomy experiences them to some extent. Without a prostate, of course, there is no ejaculation during the male orgasm, but the orgasm itself is unaffected as it is triggered by impulses from the brain.

Another option to be considered was radioactive seeding of the prostate or brachytherapy. Its advantage is that there is no surgery involved and therefore the risk of impotence and incontinence are less. However, damage to other tissues and organs can occur as a side effect, and the technique may not be as effective in eliminating the cancer as removing the organ surgically. On the other hand, if the cancer has spread beyond the prostate, the radiation may still eliminate it, as the radiation covers a larger area than just the prostate.

The third option my urologist presented was the "watchful waiting" approach. The idea here is that as the cancer may never spread beyond the prostate or only do so later in life, why risk the consequences of surgery now? The status and progress of the disease is watched carefully, monitored by regular PSA tests. For men with small, moderately aggressive cancers that appear to be localized within the prostate, like mine appeared to be, 40 percent will have cancer in their bones in 10 years; 70 percent will have bone cancer by 15 years. These are not good statistics if one is planning on living more than 10 more years.

I learned that in young men in their 40's and 50's, prostate cancer spreads faster than in older men because it is fed by higher levels of testosterone. As the levels decline with age, so does the rate of spread of prostate cancer. Because of my age, I rejected the "watchful waiting" option. Had I been 70 or 80 years old, it might have held some promise. In fact, many men die with prostate cancer although not from it. It simply progresses slowly in older men while other diseases and/or disabilities catch up with them. Because of this, the American Cancer Society (1999) suggests that men over 75 might not benefit from annual PSA testing.

Dr. Stonehouse recommended surgery because of my age. I was healthy enough to recover well and my cancer seemed to be contained. For both reasons I did not choose radiation therapy. I went along with my doctor's recommendation. I wanted to eliminate the cancer if at all possible and achieve a cure. I agreed with my doctor and with Patrick Walsh both of whom felt that a radical prostatectomy was the treatment of choice for a young person my age whose cancer appeared curable. If I chose to wait, the cancer could spread and I might miss my opportunity for a complete cure.

Dr. Stonehouse preferred what is known as a "retropubic radical prostatectomy." This means that an incision is made in the lower abdomen between the navel and the pubic bone through which the prostate removal is conducted. The alternative method, a "perineal radical prostatectomy," involves making the initial incision in the skin between the scrotum and anus. There are advantages and disadvantages to each and Patrick Walsh discusses them in his book. Robotic surgery, the DaVinci method for removing the prostate, is now available and may be an improvement over open radical prostatectomy because it is less invasive and the recovery time is faster, but the long-term statistics to evaluate it are not yet available.

Some, such as Dr. William Catalona, Senior Medical Editor of the Urological Research Foundation, St. Louis and presently of Northwestern Memorial Hospital, Chicago, feel that the DaVinci method is less preferred because the robotic arm lacks the "human touch" and it is not possible to feel the prostate gland and evaluate it as a surgeon does with his fingers. Dr. Catalona expresses his views of DaVinci robotics in his Quest newsletter (Catalona, 2006).

We scheduled my surgery for six weeks hence—August 13th. In the meantime, I was told, I had to donate three pints of my own blood to be used, if necessary, to replace blood lost in the operation. This was not a pleasant thought—that I was going to be doing three pints worth of bleeding during the whole affair! The three separate donations at the Red Cross center were required to be completed at least one week prior to my surgery. I had planned on running in the Empire State Games on July 26th which meant that I would have to start my donations the week before the Games in order to be done in time for my surgery. In fact, I would have to give my first pint five days before competing!

8

The Empire State Games

The Games went off as scheduled on July 26th and 27th, but my performances were mediocre. My 100 meter time was slower than I had hoped for—13.62 seconds, the equivalent of a 13.4 by hand timing; I had run 13.3 in the Senior Games earlier in the summer. In the 200 meters, I stumbled coming out of the starting blocks and finished at 28.16 seconds, slower than the 27.3 run a few weeks before. Two relays, 4x100 meters and 4x400 meters, resulted in a stiffened left knee, a bruised right heel and a slight pull of the right quadriceps. Did the loss of a pint of blood a few days earlier predispose me to injury? To decreased performance? Or, had I simply overtrained as the summer progressed? My experience as a masters runner has taught me that it becomes easier to overtrain as one ages. The intensity and duration of workouts one was able to handle five years ago, now produce an overtrained or injured athlete. Knowing when to scale back the workouts to accommodate an ageing physiology becomes imperative as one moves into their 40's and 50's. I have been overtrained through these years more often than I have been undertrained, and seldom have I achieved the peak performances I thought I was capable of. Running well and doing so consistently is an art—the art of knowing one's ageing physical capacity and what the mind is revealing as to how the body feels. If I am tired today is it because I have pushed harder than I ought to have earlier in the week? Or is it because of other factors related to my work and family that I am tired? Often, it is difficult to evaluate the source of such feelings. Now, more than ever, I choose to err on the side of added rest. I prefer the expression "less is better" to "no pain, no gain."

No serious runner would think of donating a pint of blood five days prior to competition. The loss of red blood cells at that time would not be compensated rapidly enough by added production in order to restore the blood to its prior level. Oxygen uptake would be affected and with decreases in speed and/or endurance resulting. I had little choice, however, if I wanted to proceed with my surgery scheduled for two-and-one-half weeks after the Games.

Prostate cancer, in its early stages, does not result in impaired physical activity. Nor may there be any indication that something is not right. It is precisely at this time that detection is important. If symptoms begin to appear, the disease may be spreading and it may be too late to cure it. I ran my best times when, ignorant of the cancer I carried around with me, my disease was present, but undetected. Prostate cancer is very prevalent, even in younger men. For this reason, men over 40, in my opinion, ought to be tested regularly for prostate cancer with a PSA test.

9

Carpe Diem

My son, Will, and three of his friends, at my urging, had formed a 4x100 meter relay team and had won their event in the 9–10 year-old age group in the local Hershey Track and Field meet for kids. I was their coach and we worked on baton passes and conditioning every week. The state meet was to be held the weekend in Waterloo, New York following the meeting that Beth and I had with my urologist. An activity that would normally have been foremost in my mind and eagerly anticipated, was now supplanted by the somber medical news I had recently received. It would have been easy to tell Will that, under the circumstances, Dad's illness would not allow us to travel to Waterloo that weekend. Yet, I was not about to allow my current predicament to overshadow other important aspects of mine or my family's lives. Again, as with the trip to the Zoo, it was not what I wanted to do at the time, but I felt I had to honor the commitment made to Will and his teammates, not just because I had agreed to coach the boys in the state meet, but because my own state of mind depended on it. When faced with a potentially terminal illness, it is important to maintain a semblance of normalcy in the rest of one's life, for that is the matrix within which we function. Whether we realize it or not, what gives meaning to each day is the complex web or network of interrelationships defined by work, home, family, church, friends and acquaintances within which we live, move and have our being. I know of one person who when informed he had prostate cancer, refused to go to work, answer telephone calls at home or provide well meaning friends with any information about his condition, other than he was "presently unavailable."

A good friend, Brenda, who, when informed she had kidney cancer and that her left kidney had to come out, responded this way: "Before I went into the hospital I was so scared I went out for lobster dinners three nights in a row. I did everything to plan my death so if I died everything would be O.K. Once I did that I was truly able to relax. I took pictures of what I wanted each person to receive and labeled them. I did all kinds of things. For me, I had to deal with my mortality before I could deal with anything else. I was really, really scared." She continued, "Maybe you are lucky and not so scared, but I think men don't allow themselves to think about fear. Or, they feel they have to hold up a mask that says—I'm macho; I don't get scared. Anytime anyone has to have surgery, especially when you haven't had much before, it is very scary."

My reply to Brenda, the week before my surgery, went like this: "I guess I am really not very scared. At least I don't feel scared or have any anxiety. A lot of people have been praying for me and that is a big help, I am sure. Also, I have been using Silva Mind Control methods—positive affirmations at Alpha level, and some personal healing, so I feel I am doing something about my state of health prior to the surgery that should make it go better, and maybe even reduce the cancer. That is my intent, anyway. Other than that, I go about life in the normal way, meeting work responsibilities, doing things with the kids and experiencing life in general. I make a conscious effort to live in the present and not allow the disease (which in a sense is my enemy) to interfere with my regular living in any way. I enjoy life—why should I allow the cancer to disrupt my life when I enjoy living in the first place? By making this effort I avoid harmful thinking about various scenarios that could conceivably happen, but probably won't. After it is all over, I would kick myself for wasting all that time worrying. So why worry about it to begin with? I am also taking responsibility for my illness by reading up on prostate cancer so that I can ask intelligent questions of my doctor and feel like a participant in my treatment rather than just letting him tell me what to do. This also avoids building up scenarios in my mind that could happen, but most likely won't (worry) because I know medically what can happen and what cannot.

This is what works for me. I am in a good state of mind. I am not possessed with worry. I am enjoying the days for what they offer rather than having them ruined by anxiety about what could happen in the future. I will let the future happen, then deal with it when it is here. In the meantime, I am doing all I can to enjoy my work, my family, my kids and it is happening. My prognosis is good for a cure because this cancer has apparently been caught early. At least all indications now suggest that that is true. I am content in that hope. For now, it will do until I know more. I like my urologist and have confidence in him; we have gotten good reports about him from others too. My approach is quite different from yours, but like you it is working for me. I often wondered if I ever got into a situation like this, how I would respond to it."

Beth and I had chosen to be open with others about my disease. We talked to Katie and Will about it once I had been given the bone scan results and we knew to the fullest extent possible what we were dealing with. We have always been honest and forthright with our children. They were able to understand why Dad was seeing the special doctor and why he had to go into the hospital for an operation soon. We used the word "cancer" in describing my condition.

I received many cards and letters from friends that were uplifting. Had I been reclusive and inhibited over sharing what I knew with others, I would not have benefited from their outpouring of care not only in written form, but from their nurturing thoughts and prayers.

Through a family friend I located an internet group full of information on prostate cancer—the Johns Hopkins prostate cancer listserve. Through the many daily email reports, so much I couldn't read it all, from others like myself, doctors and prostate cancer survivors I learned the details of others' experiences with the disease. There are many treatments for prostate cancer—some unproven and at the frontiers of research, some standard and accepted like those I mentioned, and some unorthodox that fall into the category of holistic medicine. Saw palmetto and vitamin supplements, for example, are among the latter. Some would consider prayer and Silva Mind control as forms of holistic medicine.

My son and his relay teamates competed in the Hershey's state meet. I was there as their coach. They were timed in 70.1 seconds for the 4x100 meter relay and received second place ribbons among 9 and 10 year olds for their efforts. The boys and I had worked hard to get ready for the meet.

We were rewarded for our efforts. When a deadly disease pays us a visit, one needs such sources of enjoyment and satisfaction to counterbalance the negativity that is otherwise omnipresent.

10

Surgery

Several days before my surgery on the 13th, Dr. Stonehouse called to see how I was getting along, to confirm that I was ready to proceed as planned with the prostatectomy, and to remind me that the day before on the 12th I was due at the hospital for pre-admission tests. The actual surgery was scheduled for 7:30 a.m. and I was to check into the hospital at 6:30 a.m. I was told not to drink any water the morning of the surgery, but when the day came, forgot this admonition and downed a glass or two, as is my custom, upon waking. Water in the stomach could work its way back up and into the lungs if I was to regurgitate under anaesthesia as sometimes happens. Since the anaesthesia was to be administered only a short time after I had awakened, it was an important order to follow. If I was to swallow water, the surgery could be postponed.

I was also asked to consider an important question. If my cancer had spread beyond the prostate, into nearby tissues, and this would be determined by a lymph node biopsy, then the prostatectomy would be aborted. In which case, my surgeon would need to follow a different course of action. Removal of the prostate would serve no useful purpose if the cancer was elsewhere beyond the confines of the gland. The next point of attack, I was told, would have to be reduction of testosterone levels in my body. As testosterone feeds the developing cancer cells, the spread of the disease would have to be slowed down as a means of treatment. I, as well as my urologist, knew my chances—49 percent probability that the cancer was beyond the prostate, although we knew it was not in my bony structure, and according to Walsh's tables, 8 percent chance that it was in my lymph nodes. To cut the testosterone level, castration would be necessary. The question I was to consider if my lymph node biopsy was positive was whether I would prefer medical castration by removal of the testicles or chemical castration involving injections every three months for the rest of my life to block testosterone production. The latter option was associated with muscle atrophy, impotence, osteoporosis and loss of libido. As long as the surgeon had my abdominal cavity open, he could proceed with the surgical removal of my testicles if this was my choice. Otherwise, he would sew me back up and we would be done and I would begin the injections.

Beth and I checked into the hospital and I was taken to a room adjoining the one in which the operation was to take place. I was given a pair of long tight fitting stockings and a hospital gown and told to put them on. The stockings, I had learned, were to force the blood in my legs into the larger, deeper veins in my legs where the chances of a clot forming were less. Blood clots are a potential complication of this type of surgery and must be guarded against. The probability of their occurrence is highest during surgery and decreases with time after. I was placed on a portable bed and given a relaxant by injection. In a few minutes it was time to say goodbye to Beth and I was wheeled into the operating room and moved to the operating table under bright lights. I had decided to tell Dr. Stonehouse about my consumption of the forbidden water. If anything was to happen, at least my last waking act would have been an honest one. I was asked how much I had drunk and tried to remember, probably underestimating the actual amount. My doctor and his assistant conferred briefly, then indicated that the operation was to proceed. I uttered an inaudible sigh of relief. Then, I was asked what I had decided to do should the prostatectomy have to be aborted due to cancer in my lymph nodes. I replied that I had decided upon chemical castration. My reasoning was that medical castration was permanent; chemical castration was not. Advances in medicine may someday present different alternatives, and more favorable ones, to someone faced with castration to block testosterone. If by the small chance that it was necessary in my case, I wanted to be able to avail myself of the benefits of those advances. The anesthesiologist placed a mask over my face and I was asked to breathe deeply. That was the last I remembered until I regained consciousness hours later in the recovery room.

11

Benefits of Regular Exercise

My recollection of those first awakening moments remains clear, although at the time my mind was not. It was a struggle to stay conscious due to the anaesthetic that still remained in my body. I was aware that I was no longer in the operating room and that the surgery was over, and aware that something major had taken place in my abdominal region. I felt no pain and lapsed back into unconsciousness. My next recollection was that of being in the hospital room that I was to call home for several days. Beth was standing alongside my bed. I cannot remember her exact words, but she held my hand and assured me that the surgery had been performed and that all had gone well. I noted that it was now after 1:00 p.m.

In my absence she and her good friend, Marsha, had been in the waiting room. Dr. Stonehouse had been in to report on my condition after surgery while I was still in the recovery room. He assured her that the surgery had been successful, the prostate gland and seminal vesicles had been removed, and that my "margins were clear," meaning that the cancer appeared to have been confined to the prostate. In addition, he was visibly impressed with my degree of fitness. It seems that most men he sees in their 50's have their small capillaries plugged, but mine were wide open. When he had made his initial incision, the blood had spouted up like a geyser, quite unusual in older men, and much more typical of youth. I knew I was physically fit and healthy. What was interesting was that someone could look inside my body and come to the same conclusion. It only verified that my active lifestyle was producing healthy results.

You see, there is a cost to be paid for inactivity as we grow older. If the smallest blood vessels are not used, they become non-functional. What then happens to the tissues they feed? Part of the function of the circulatory system is to remove waste products from the body. Who would opt for a less than efficient system of tissue maintenance? Many men and women do, though, by their choice of a sedentary lifestyle.

In the same vein, when Beth and I had received the results of my bone scan, Dr. Stonehouse had noted that I had no evidence of arthritis and that most men my age have at least some. Of course, I knew that—I didn't need a bone scan to tell me. It was again interesting and satisfying, however, to have the x-ray machine confirm another aspect of my good overall state of health.

From an evolutionary standpoint, we humans need regular exercise. Our bodies evolved with a regimen of hard physical daily work. Our species is around 6 million years old (Holden, 2000; Galik et al. 2004) and still possesses traits that evolved under and were beneficial to a lifestyle quite different from that of today's Homo sapiens. The lack of physical activity in the lives of people today has contributed to a society in which most people are overweight and have a variety of other afflictions that can at least in part be attributed to inactivity: high blood pressure and high cholesterol levels, artherosclerosis, type-2 diabetes, mental stress, and muscle and bone degeneration in old age. Physical inactivity is now the third leading cause of death in the United States and contributes to the second leading cause, obesity, according to the Center for Disease Control and Prevention. Dr. William Catalona has researched the effects of obesity upon prostate cancer aggressiveness and reports positive links in his recent Quest newsletter (Catalona, 2007). Obese men were significantly more likely to have a biopsy Gleason score of greater than 6, a higher percentage of cancer in the biopsy specimen and a greater proportion of extracapsular tumor extension, i.e., cancer cells that had spread outside of the prostatic capsule. Currently, more than 60 percent of adults in the United States are overweight and 30 percent are obese. The latter number is expected to reach 40 percent by 2010. We cannot just turn off those genes that took millions of years to evolve.

In studies of exercising adults, Booth and Neufer (2005) report that increased activity level of skeletal muscle modulates a range of genes that produce dramatic physiological effects including, for example, limiting the rise of blood glucose after the next meal by making insulin work better in moving glucose into muscle. It is estimated that the average hunter-gatherer expended about 1,000 kilocalories per day in physical activity while consuming 3,000 kilocalories, a ratio of 3:1 for energy consumed/expended. Today's typical sedentary person consumes about 2,400 kilocalories per day while expending 300 kilocalories in physical activity, a ratio of 8:1. The obesity epidemic we see today is grounded not so much in overeating as it is in lack of exercise. From an evolutionary viewpoint, to choose not to exercise regularly and vigorously is unhealthy. In fact, according to recent studies by Utah biomechanics expert, Dennis Bramble, and physical anthropologist, Daniel Lieberman, the human body exhibits specialized adaptations in muscles, tendons and bones for endurance running that developed 2 million years ago in the genus <u>Homo</u>, possibly to become better scavengers on the African savanna (Bramble and Lieberman, 2004).

Dr. Ralph Paffenbarger of Harvard University conducted a study between 1975 and 1992 of 13,485 Harvard alumni males of average age 57.5 years, and found that regular, vigorous exercise significantly lengthens life span. For every hour of vigorous exercise, a person's life is extended by two to three hours, on the average. Over the lifetime of a 75-year-old man, as much as two years of extended life span may be gained by those who have a recent history of regular exercise. In his study, the greater the energy that was expended in regular exercise, the longer the men lived. Vigorous activity produced extra longevity, but light, moderate activity did not. Therefore, those who run, swim, cycle or engage in other physical activity can expect to live longer because of it. The same study also showed that inactivity and an overweight condition were as detrimental to long life as vigor was beneficial (Lee and Paffenbarger, 2000).

Research at the Salk Institute suggests that an active life, either physically or mentally, can have a positive impact on the brain. Regular running and intensive mental exercise associated with an enriched environment in mice have been shown to improve learning and promote the growth of new neurons as well as synaptic plasticity in a part of the brain called the hippocampus, important to the formation of new memories (Kemperman et al., 1997; van Praag et al., 1999, 2002). Since mice and humans are both mammals the assumption is that the brains of both may respond similarly to a common stimulus.

Likewise, mice given an enriched environment in which exercise and toys replaced standard laboratory cages had less buildup of beta-amyloid plaques which have been associated with Alzheimer's disease (Lazarov et al., 2005). Indeed, some epidemiological studies on humans have suggested the same, i.e., that exercise, education and intellectually challenging activities diminish the risk of Alzheimer's disease.

12

Hospital Recovery

My recovery progressed as Dr. Stonehouse said that it would. My good health would support the healing process. During the surgery, the three pints of my blood I had donated were used. Receiving one's own blood is better than receiving another person's even if it is the same blood type. When one has enough advance notice of their surgery, and when blood may be required to replace that lost, putting one's own blood into storage for later use is recommended. Blood is scarce to begin with and post-surgery healing is enhanced by the perfect match between a person and their own blood.

On the evening of the day of my prostatectomy, my nurse got me out of bed for a walk. As difficult as this was, it is done to promote recovery. Walking improves blood flow to the surgical wound area. For prostate surgery patients it is recommended as a daily practice beginning immediately following surgery and continuing through the at-home healing period.

In order to walk, however, I had to carry my plastic bag of reddish-tinged urine which was connected to my penis by a Foley catheter tube, push my IV stand in front of me which was on wheels, and all the while use care that I did not dislodge another plastic balloon of fluid that hung from a tube coming out of a hole in my abdomen. As I was not able to move very rapidly, this was not as difficult as it sounds. Since the bladder had been cut and reformed around the urethra, it could not yet function independently. The catheter tube had been inserted while I was under anesthesia, as had the tube in my lower abdomen which drained the internal surgical wound region. A nurse periodically checked and drained the plastic balloon and the catheter bag.

I spent three days and part of a fourth in the hospital. My best experience was being able to walk around the floor I was on at will. Always the runner, I paced off the distance of "one lap" so I knew how many times around the perimeter of the floor constituted a mile. On the second day post-surgery I walked a total of one and one-quarter miles. I had rapidly become semi-skilled in pushing my IV stand while watching where I was headed and keeping my two bags of waste fluids in the proper position for comfort and safety. Oh, yes, and then also keeping my hospital gown proper to prevent inadvertent indecent exposure.

Our neighbor, Debbie, was the nurse-in-charge for my floor and did me a great favor for which I will always be grateful. She secured me a private room at no extra charge. People go into hospitals for a reason—they are not well. While ordinarily I would have welcomed the company—to be at less than full health and then to have to experience someone else's ill health in close proximity—now it was that sort of sociability I was eager to forego.

The worst experience while in the hospital was not being awakened at night for pain control shots in my bottom or the bland diet I was put on, but the fact that I could not get comfortable on the bed. It was hard and induced a dull ache that would not go away no matter which way I moved. There was little room for maneuvering as I was forced to lie on my back all the time due to the location of my surgical wounds. I finally resolved the matter by buying an inflatable mattress which fit under the sheet.

My legs were still encased in tight fitting stockings which extended to my upper thighs and each leg was wrapped in a device which provided gentle mechanical massage. Again, this was to minimize chances of blood clotting. My legs were to be kept elevated when I was not walking.

I was instructed in performing "kegels," simple exercises designed to strengthen the sphincter muscle that closes off the reformed bladder. That muscle can be strengthened and thus becomes better at shutting down the flow of urine, important to regaining continence. A friend who underwent the same operation advised me to do kegels as often as I was able to. I performed the kegels according to my doctor's advice, which was less often. It seemed that one could overwork the sphincter muscle just as one could, with a lack of discretion, overwork any other muscle in the body.

I had hopes that I would be able to leave the hospital and go home at the earliest date three days following surgery. In order for this to happen, I had to have clearing of the fluid in the small plastic balloon, stable vital signs, a bowel movement, and be up and walking several times a day. By the third day I was, in fact, walking seven to eight times and was covering an estimated one and one-quarter miles on my loop circuit around the hospital floor. All my signs were positive. The morning of the fourth day I was told I could go home. I was discharged at 11:00 a.m. Beth helped me into the front seat of our Toyota and in a few short minutes we were pulling into our driveway.

13

A Major Jolt

While at home, the walking continued. Dr. Stonehouse indicated to me that the more walking I was able to do, the more rapid would be my healing. After a day or two of walking back-and-forth inside the house, I strapped a leg bag on and headed outside. Before leaving the hospital I had been instructed by a nurse as to how to substitute the large plastic catheter bag that I had to hand-carry for the smaller bag that strapped to my thigh beneath a pair of loose-fitting pants. I was to wear a catheter bag for three weeks at which time the catheter could be removed and I would handle my incontinence with disposable absorbent inserts that fit inside my underwear.

A great joy of each day, very soon after returning home, became my daily walks in the neighborhood. I had a fixed course I followed in the morning, at mid-day and in the evening which increased from three-fourths to one-and-three-fourths miles as my healing progressed. As early as a week-and-a-half after my hospital discharge I was walking five miles a day. As time went along and I felt better, I would challenge myself to complete the course in less time than before. This was probably not in the best interests of my recovery, as my body let me know several times that I had overdone it. Aside from some overindulgence in my walking routine, I experienced little pain. As long as I did not try to force the issue, I required no pain medicine during the healing process. Perhaps I was fortunate in this regard. It is not everyone's experience.

When I was not walking, I was lying or sitting in bed with legs up as I had been instructed to do. I still wore the tight stockings, but these were discarded after a few days. I required a daily nap and continued to take one even after I returned to work part-time. Regaining full strength following a prostatectomy is a gradual process that takes some time, more so for some men than others. My minister recently had the same surgery and reported to me that three months afterwards 85 percent of his strength had returned, but that he still required a daily nap.

During my convalescence, mental concentration was tiring, especially in the days following surgery and even extending up until my return to work. This was particularly the case while in the hospital. I appreciated visits from friends, but easily tired, especially when I had to "make conversation." Those who overstayed their visit, frankly, were more of a burden than any help to me.

The close correspondence between my physical and mental states was made even clearer to me while at home. Although recovering, I found even the demands of normal conversation with my wife, Beth, to be difficult and wearying at times. She, who performed nobly in the role of parent, wife and care-giver, deserved more than I was capable of giving her in terms of ready conversation and attention to her needs. I felt like an old sponge, trying, but failing to absorb all that came my way, and not giving much intellectually, or emotionally, in return. Our two bouncing, bounding children, although loved much, were often more than I could handle as I was unable to match the level of energy and enthusiasm that they radiated. The feelings of frustration felt over the difficulty of close interpersonal relationships that had heretofore been enjoyable and entered into with ease only compounded my sense of physical and mental dislocation during these early weeks following surgery. Even after returning to work, I was not the usual vigorous, energetic soul that I had been earlier that summer. A radical prostatectomy serves up a major jolt to one's body, and is felt both physically and mentally and for some time afterwards.

14

Pathology Results

The day after my catheter was removed I went back to work. I also stopped doing the kegels as they now seemed not to benefit me much. They seemed to me to be more of a nuisance and something that was easier to dispense with than to continue doing even though they were simple to perform and any doctor would have instructed me otherwise. I had control over my urinary stream, but was leaking. The absorbent pads solved that problem. I had been advised not to drive a car, to avoid strenuous exercise and to not lift heavy objects prior to three weeks post-surgery. I later learned that these precautions would prevent the possible tearing open of an incision by a sudden jerk to hit the car brake or by the strain of a heavy lift. I adhered to these rules, but found that with the catheter out I was more mobile. I started driving to work and back and experienced little difficulty. Initially, I went back to work half-time. I still napped in the afternoon and needed the extra rest it provided. My walks continued, but the venue was now a cemetery in the neighborhood of my workplace. I began teaching fall classes two days after returning to work. I was a week late for the beginning of the fall term and colleagues had filled in for me in the meantime. At five weeks post-surgery I returned to work full-time. My five miles per day of walking continued, but the afternoon nap seemed unnecessary now.

One week after surgery, Beth and I returned to my urologist's office for discussion of the surgery, removal of my surgical staples and to receive the pathology results from tests done on the excised prostate gland. We were told that when the prostate and seminal vesicles were removed, both neurovascular bundles had been saved. It is standard practice to remove the seminal vesicles along with the prostate since they are a "conduit" for transmission of the cancer to the bloodstream. Saving the nerve bundles that control erections had positive implications for recovery of sexual potency. However, the pathologist found that the cancer had not been confined to the right side of my prostate. The margins were confirmed to be negative as my doctor had observed during the surgery, but there was cancer in both lobes, not just one. The right lobe was 10–20 percent (by volume) cancerous and the left lobe, 5–10 percent cancerous. Neither the biopsy nor the ultrasound had found the cancer in the left lobe. Thus I was given a "false negative" with regard to the left lobe. Sometimes cancer is present in the prostate, but not detectable by biopsy and associated ultrasound. The PSA test had indicated its possible presence, but the fact that both lobes were cancerous meant that my Gleason score was really an eight and my clinical staging was T2c, indicating a more aggressive and more serious cancer than originally thought. With the different staging, Walsh's tables now indicated that the probability that the cancer was confined to the prostate had been only 22 percent. The pathology results furthermore indicated that the cancer appeared to have been contained. I had beaten the odds!

15

Return to Running

I began running again at six weeks to the date, post-surgery. At this time I was back to working my usual 9:00 a.m. to 6:00 p.m. day with a break in the middle. My doctor had advised me to wait at least six weeks before getting back into jogging. Before this, I had not felt ready to take this next step in my recovery. The energy level was not sufficient, nor had I healed enough internally to accommodate the added stress of slow running. At six weeks, however, I was ready to substitute running for the time-consuming five miles of walking per day. It had been two months since I last completed a running workout. After a layoff of this amount, considerable muscle mass and tone are lost as well as cardiovascular efficiency and to regain one's conditioning is a slow process. Returning to the physical level of activity accustomed to prior to surgery should be undertaken with caution. "Letting one's body be the guide" is probably the best advice to give as each person will recover from surgery at a different rate and be able to resume running according to the uniqueness of their own body type and physiology. If a slow, short run feels good, then it is probably a sign that the body will accommodate a slightly higher intensity or duration of workout. Care should be taken at the start, however, not to attempt to increase the level of workouts at too great a rate beyond what is comfortable. It is tempting to use one's level of pre-surgery workout performance as the guide to resuming training. This can be a mistake and should be guarded against as internal healing of a longer-term nature must now occur simultaneously with the resumption of physical activity. The former may place limits on the extent to which the latter may be realized. A return to the level of pre-surgery performance may be a long-term goal, but resumption of training following surgery for the masters athlete should be governed by the short-term standard of doing what feels right and is comfortable.

My first run was a mile-and-a-half jog along the streets near the College where I worked. In the locker room I weighed myself at 156 pounds, down from my normal 166 prior to surgery. The run had gone well and although there had been leakage, the disposable pad did its job. The following day I resumed weight training, in much modified form and with lighter weights compared to what I had been doing six or more weeks ago. I had muscle mass to rebuild, and physical endurance to regain, but I had at least begun that process, and it felt good, like seeing an old friend again.

Over the following month I gradually brought my 5K time on the track down to under 27 minutes and turned some 400m's in the mid-80 second range. For me, this was comfortable. My continence was improving gradually. I got to the point where the jarring of running no longer produced wet shorts. After a month of running and at 10 weeks post-surgery I dispensed with the absorbent pads. Yet, it was still occasionally the case that some slight wetting would occur, usually after bending over or upon coughing, but it was not enough to bring back the pads nor enough to be outwardly noticeable. Today, my continence is for all practical purposes normal, with only infrequent minor incidents. The return to running, by strengthening pelvic muscles, probably hastened the return to full continence.

One particular result of the surgery that does have its lingering effect is that of a smaller bladder capacity. Due to the bladder having been cut and reformed during surgery its original volume has been reduced. This means that somewhat more frequent urination is required and the urge to do so is experienced more often. Although not a problem when restroom facilities are present, I now, in addition, need to anticipate the possibility of awkward situations arising where facilities might be hard to find. A little forethought is usually all that is required to forestall an embarrassing moment.

The need to anticipate such situations was driven home to me when in Costa Rica for a conference in 1997. I took a morning bus tour that involved a three hour ride through the mountains. Not mindful of my somewhat reduced bladder capacity, I enjoyed my breakfast including coffee and orange juice, then promptly got on the bus which had no restroom. It was not long before the jostling of the bus on the mountain roads and my lack of foresight regarding liquids at breakfast produced extreme bladder duress. Finally, when I could stand it no longer I got up from my seat, explained the urgency of the situation to the bus driver, and asked him to stop the bus. He pulled over understandingly, I got out, and dashed into the trees and undergrowth by the side of the road where I promptly relieved myself. After what seemed like an eternity, I returned to the bus greatly embarrassed, thanked the driver, and while trying not to look at the other passengers, returned to my seat and we drove off. A lesson was learned.

16

Side Effects

After my prostate was removed, I was given another PSA test, while still in the hospital, to determine if any cancer cells were growing anywhere and contributing to a rise in blood antigen specific to prostate cancer. That test, as well as others taken since to October, 2001, had all been negative, i.e., a level of PSA less than 0.1 ng/ml, or basically undetectable. As of October, 2001, over five years had passed since my surgery, and there was no indication of any prostate cancer remaining. I continued to take PSA tests along with digital rectal exams at six month intervals, to monitor myself for the presence of cancer as well as for recovery from surgery. The digital rectal exam continues to be given as a means of monitoring the surgical area to be sure that no abnormal growths are occurring. My October, 2001 PSA test showed a level of 0.2 ng/ml, within the statistical error, viz., 0.1 ng/ml for that level of reading. Although my urologist was not concerned about the slight increase in PSA, he asked me to come back in three months to repeat the test. The PSA test is currently the most reliable and accepted method among urologists for monitoring the status of prostate cancer in patients.

Many men fear prostate surgery because of the potential complications of incontinence and impotence. In my experience, the incontinence was only very temporary and is now a part of my past. Recovery of sexual potency takes longer, however, and proceeds more slowly. There may never be complete recovery to the level of what once had been. In my case, it has been more of a problem, as it has been for many men, than the incontinence. Orgasms are just as common as before and that is to be expected as they are centered in the brain. Erectile dysfunction continues to be a factor in my recovery, but there seems to be some slow progress, and there are many treatments now available to deal with it. Viagra is the most promising and effective of these, in my opinion, after having tried several of the others. New drugs that operate in different ways from Viagra, such as Levitra and Cialis, have emerged and new ones are continually under development and will soon arrive on pharmacists's shelves. I have a friend who is an ethnobotanist working with an Indian tribe in the Amazon. He relates that the men have their own "Viagra"—a mixture of chili peppers, termite heads and ants! Natural product chemists will work to discover the active ingredient and synthesize it so pharmaceutical companies can put it into a prescription drug for you and I. Or, do you prefer the real thing?

17

Recurrence

My last PSA test in April, 2001 had yielded <0.1 ng PSA/ml. I was approaching five years post-surgery with no change in PSA. Dr. Stonehouse assured me that I was "probably" cured. Five years of PSA tests at <0.1 was enough for him to feel very confident that the surgery and follow-up had produced the desired cure, i.e., the cancer was removed and would not return. Only in a very small percentage of men, he told me, does it return after five years. Thus it was that I approached my next six-month PSA testing with a sense that any serious cancer monitoring was behind me. Of course I had to be tested and this would continue as a formality for the rest of my life. What I had been through was over and finished now. It was all a done deal.

Such was my outlook as I went to my urologist's office in early November, 2001 to receive the results of the latest PSA test, this one at 5 years, 2 months post-surgery. It had come back at 0.2 ng/ml, higher than usual for me, but still not enough to get alarmed over. I was told that statistically there was no difference between 0.2 and <0.1. A PSA of 0.2 would still be considered negligible. Dr. William J. Catalona, who established the rules for PSA testing back in 1991, considers any PSA value less than 0.3 ng/ml as negligible because of the difficulty of detecting PSA in assays at this level. Thus, a value of 0.2 ng/ml or 0.1 ng/ml would be considered essentially zero.

It was recommended that I return for a re-test in 3 months. That would provide a check of the October testing. Since I had never had a PSA test come back at 0.2 ng/ml since my surgery, I was mildly concerned. Thus it was that I returned in early January, 2002 to learn that my PSA level had risen to 0.3 ng/ml. This was enough for Dr. Stonehouse to tell me that I was possibly seeing some prostate regrowth—some small piece of the original prostate had not been removed at the time of my surgery and now had grown to the point that it was producing measurable PSA. Alternatively, even though I had had clear margins when my prostate was removed, some small extracapsular extension of the cancer may have gone undetected. Because there was no way to validate which of these two explanations accounted for my rising PSA, or if both were involved, radiation treatment for cancer was being prescribed and I was referred to a radiation oncologist. Several names were mentioned, neither of which meant anything to me and I chose one because his office was near to my workplace. I later learned that I had made an excellent choice, that the oncologist I picked, Dr. Joseph Abraham, was experienced and had a fine reputation. An appointment was made for me to meet with him in early February. Dr. Stonehouse, in the meantime, wanted my PSA level re-tested and so this was done a month after the 0.3 ng/ml reading and I tested out at a PSA level of 0.4 ng/ml. Thus, I had gone from 0.2 to 0.4 ng/ml in the space of four months.

The news of my recurrence was a shock, but it was not as difficult to deal with emotionally as had the initial cancer diagnosis been 5 ½ years ago. Beth had known of my doctor's appointment and so I called her with the news—"I have another chapter to write for my book." She knew right away what that meant.

18

Dr. Joseph Abraham, Radiation Oncologist

Beth and I went together to the scheduled appointment with my radiation oncologist, Dr. Abraham. The PSA test result of 0.4 ng/ml had not come back yet from my urologist's lab, so the consultation was based on 0.3 ng/ml being the most recent PSA test. In his office we talked of my condition and probable diagnosis. It was probable that I was having a recurrence of the cancer. However, a PSA level of 0.3 ng/ml could also mean that some benign tissue was left behind following surgery and it was growing back. Apparently, there is not a lot of evidence for this latter effect, but it is given as an interpretation of a low, but rising PSA level.

We discussed external beam radiation treatment, how it is conducted and its side effects. For my condition with a PSA = 0.3 ng/ml, nutritional therapy was recommended and I was advised to read Dr. Charles E. "Snuffy" Myers, Jr.'s 2000 book, Eating Your Way to Better Health— The Prostate Forum Nutrition Guide, which describes a number of nutritional supplements and dietary recommendations that have been found to be effective against prostate cancer. Dr. Myers is Professor of Medicine and Urology and Cancer Center Director at the University of Virginia in Charlottesville. I was cautioned, however, that if I was going to undergo radiation therapy not to wait too long to begin it. If the PSA rises over 1.0, then the cancer may be too large in size for the radiation prescribed to kill the innermost cells of the carcinoma. A higher dosage in this event might cause undue damage to healthy tissues. Therefore, radiation therapy is felt to be most effective when the cancerous area is small, i.e., as would be true, for example, for a PSA of 0.4–0.6 ng/ml. If nutritional therapy was successful for me and my PSA level dropped or did not increase, then I may not need radiation therapy. However, were my PSA level to rise to 0.5 ng/ml, then it likely would not be working and I would be advised to elect radiation therapy as the preferred treatment. The nutritional therapy was worth trying at this point, I was told. In the meantime, continued PSA testing would document the cancer's progress. As radiation therapy has some adverse side effects, it was not to be undertaken unless there was good cause to use it.

Hormonal therapy was also mentioned, and some doctors, as various web sites will attest, recommend hormonal therapy along with radiation therapy when PSA levels rise after radical prostatectomy. Dr. Abraham was not of the view that both should be used together at this time because reducing testosterone causes men to lose bone and muscle mass, lose their sex drive and put on weight, all serious side effects, although they are reversible when the hormonal treatments stop. In his view, advances in radiation therapy protocol have progressed to the point where a maximally effective dose of x-rays may be delivered to the prostate bed over an optimal period of time with side effects minimized to the greatest extent possible. This has been due to the administering of radiation to a large number of prostate cancer patients over a long period and refining the methods used to obtain the best effects. In his estimation, hormonal therapy with its more extreme health risks should be reserved for advanced cases where radiation therapy has already been tried.

In search of more information, I visited the web site of The Brady Urological Institute at Johns Hopkins. Here, I learned that about 35 percent of men who have had their prostates removed had a rise in their PSA levels in the 10 years following surgery. In fact, Patrick Walsh and his colleagues (Pound et al., 1999) compiled 10,000 patient years of data from a follow-up study of 1,997 men between 1982–97 which they used to produce a chart showing the risk of developing metastatic prostate cancer, or cancer that has spread to other parts of the body, in men who have recurrence following surgery. The chart is based on the Gleason score for the removed prostate (whether your score is 5–7 or 8–10), the time from surgery to a rise in PSA level (whether greater or less than two years), and the time in months for a doubling of PSA to occur (whether greater or less than 10 months). If the Gleason score is 8–10, then the PSA doubling time is not used. For my condition, with a Gleason score of 8 and a time to recurrence of 5 years, the chart predicted that I had a 77 percent chance of not developing metastases in three years, a 60 percent chance in five years and a 47 percent chance in seven years. Of course, this assumes that the cancer is not cured and runs its course which for some men may require many years or it may not spread at all. It is the policy of Johns Hopkins not to treat men with prostate cancer recurrence until symptoms develop, a view different from that of my radiation oncologist.

Dr. Joseph Abraham feels that prostate cancer can be cured with radiation therapy in some of the men who have recurrence after surgery and his own statistics bear this out. If the PSA level goes up after surgery, then PSA is being produced somewhere in the body. Its location could be the prostate bed or the area where the prostate was removed, a likely source, or it could have spread to the bones or via the bloodstream to a distant point in the body, or both. The actual site of the cancer cannot be known until the PSA rises to at least 2.0 or greater because scan tests that would be used are not sufficiently sensitive to detect cancer in such an early stage of development. Yet, if one were to wait until the cancer was large enough to be detectable as to location, it would be far less treatable. The Johns Hopkins data suggests that men who had cancer in the lymph nodes or seminal vesicles at the time of surgery would very likely experience distant recurrence or metastatic cancer. For those who had extracapsular extension, about half of the recurrences occurred in the prostate bed. In these men, radiotherapy has a reasonable chance of success (Aronowitz, 2002). Johns Hopkins apparently feels that because prostate cancer develops slowly, they would subject many men to unnecessary side effects if they treated recurrence after surgery before symptoms appeared. And, the fact is that many men who experience recurrence after surgery may do very well for years just with "watchful waiting" as a treatment.

In his own work, Dr. Jesse Aronowitz of the Hill Medical Center in Syracuse followed 28 men who had recurrence following radical prostatectomy and whose PSA levels had been monitored for between one and five years (Aronowitz, 2002). Most had positive margins and about half had extracapsular extension as determined by a pathologist. The Gleason scores of the 28 were seven or higher in over half of the men. In 17 of the 28, PSA became undetectable (<0.1 ng/ml) after irradiation. The success rate was higher for those with Gleason scores less than seven. And, 2/3 of the patients whose PSA was less than 1.0 prior to radiotherapy did well, whereas only half of the patients whose PSA was greater than 1.0 did well. If PSA levels begin to rise following surgery, as mine did, the data suggests that the earlier radiotherapy is begun, the better are its chances for success. Not everyone with rising PSA's following surgery should have radiotherapy, but for patients who did not have cancer in the seminal vesicles and who still have PSA levels below 1.0 ng/ml, Dr. Aronowitz feels that there is better than 50 percent likelihood of success.

19

Eating Right

I began nutritional therapy after my first visit with Dr. Abraham. Charles Myers' book, available over his web site, was informative. Charles Myers had spent much of his life researching and recommending dietary modification as a tool in fighting prostate cancer. Then, he himself was diagnosed with prostate cancer after his wife urged him to get a PSA test. He reports on this to visitors to his web site. I learned that there are a number of foods, vitamins and minerals that may alter the development of prostate cancer. Among these are selenium, vitamins C and E, green tea, quercetin, fish oil, carotenoids, soy products, red wine, pomegranate juice and grains. Myers advocates a low fat vegan or vegetarian diet rich in vegetables, grains, cereals and fruits and fiber. Red meat should be avoided with preference being given to skinless chicken or fish. Dairy products should be minimized due to the fat they contain. For some of these recommendations there are good reasons through significant research why they affect prostate cancer. With others, their scientific validity is less substantiated.

For many years I, as well as others in my family, had been taking 500 mg of vitamin C per day. I took it because it is an antioxidant, and protects the body against hydrogen peroxide and harmful free radicals that are produced from it. In September, 2001, the month before my PSA level began rising I discontinued taking it because I wanted to see, as a trial over six months, if it made any difference to our health. I would see how many colds we contracted over this period and compare the number to our usual amount when we were on the vitamin C. I had come to question the value of my taking it each day as I had read of a negative effect in test tube studies that high doses of vitamin C could potentially promote DNA damage that could lead to cancer (Lee et al., 2001). These concerns were later put into more logical perspective by other investigators (Letters to the Editor, 2001), but at the time I had not read their opinions. Did my discontinuance of vitamin C have anything to do with my PSA rise? I may never know unless studies directly related to its effect on prostate cancer cells are done which show a causative link. Perhaps it was just a coincidence that my lack of antioxidant protection from not taking vitamin C coincided directly with my cancer recurrence or perhaps I had been unknowingly protecting myself over the past five years from the growth of a small number of cancer cells. In January, 2002 after my PSA started rising, I discontinued my family trial of vitamin C efficacy and resumed taking 500 mg of vitamin C per day.

Quercetin is a phytochemical found in many fruits and vegetables, but especially in apples. Lee et al. (2002) found that quercetin has stronger antioxidant activity than vitamin C. One hundred grams of unpeeled fresh apple—about 2/3 of a medium-sized apple—provided the antioxidant activity of 1,500 mg of vitamin C. Both vitamin C and phytochemicals are protective against cancer. The phrase, "An apple a day keeps the doctor away," seems not to be without justification.

Green tea contains antioxidants in the form of polyphenols, chemicals which have known anti-cancer activity, causing rapid shrinkage of human prostate cancers growing in mice. They do this by interfering with cell division of cancer cells. In high amounts, cancer cells are killed. Green tea may be the reason that the Chinese have low rates of prostate cancer. Myers recommends drinking plenty of it.

A nutritional supplement that Myers has researched is flax seed oil. He has observed it to have a powerful stimulant effect on the growth of prostate cancer cells in the laboratory. Yet, it is recommended as effective against prostate cancer by the University of California at Berkeley (UC Berkeley Wellness Newsletter, 2002). This is an example of the sometimes conflicting research that is to be found in the field of nutrition and cancer treatment. The Berkeley Newsletter cites a study whereby "men with prostate cancer who ate an ounce of ground flaxseeds a day as part of a low-fat diet were able to slow the progress of their cancers between the time they were diagnosed and the time of surgery." Yet, it may have been the low-fat diet and not the flax seed that was effective in this work. Flax seed contains alpha-linolenic acid which has been associated with a reduced risk of heart disease and a lowering of total blood cholesterol. Charles Myers finds that flax seed is 50 percent alpha-linolenic acid and when put on prostate cancer cells in the laboratory is a more powerful stimulus to growth than testosterone. If Myers is right, then perhaps there are better ways to lower cholesterol than by eating flax seed. After I read Myers' information, I stopped putting a product on my cereal every morning which contained large amounts of flax seed!

I have taken Charles Myers' advice on a number of foods and nutritional supplements. Those I currently am taking daily are selenium (200 mcg), vitamin E (100 International Units), lycopene (30 mg), soy milk (on my cereal), soy protein powder (30g in a fruit shake), fish oil (4000 mg), turmeric root extract (300 mg), one or more apples, a cup of green tea and 8 ounces of pomegranate juice daily. Lycopene is believed to be the active ingredient in cooked and concentrated tomato-based products which appear to help prevent and slow the growth of prostate cancer. However, a recent study in rats by Erdman and Clinton (2003) shows that eating whole tomatoes is more effective at reducing prostate cancer deaths than taking lycopene supplements. Indian curry spice turmeric contains curcumin, a polyphenol shown to be effective in inducing apoptosis in prostate cancer cells and enhancing antibody responses and modulating the immune system (Jagetia and Aggarwal, 2007; Dorai et al., 2000). Pomegranate juice has been shown to slow the rate of PSA increase following surgery or radiation (Pantuck et al., 2006). In addition, I have stopped eating red meat and only eat fish or fowl and have adhered to a low fat diet. I do not eat dairy products which means no cheese or ice cream, to my displeasure, but I have gotten used to it. I drink skim milk, however, for the calcium, but not more than one glass a day since Myers has data that indicates that too much calcium may stimulate the growth of prostate cancer. Organic skim milk costs more than regular milk, but one is assured that the cows were not fed on hormonal supplements which can then find their way into the milk product. For the most part, I began this diet in February, 2002, just after seeing Dr. Joseph Abraham for the first time and receiving his recommendation to try nutritional therapy, and continue on it today.

The American Institute for Cancer Research recommends many of the same dietary modifications as Charles Myers. In addition, they suggest eating cruciferous vegetables such as cabbage, cauliflower and broccoli, grape seed extract, and red grapes and peanuts for the resveratrol they contain, which is also found in red wine (AICR, 2002). Garlic and its organic allyl sulfur components are effective inhibitors of both prostate and stomach cancers according to the National Cancer Institute (National Cancer Institute Fact Sheet, 2005). Twenty-eight of thirty-seven observational studies on humans show cancer preventive effects of garlic, although these studies have all been epidemiological in nature or involved animal models or observations on cells in culture. None of the benefits of garlic in cancer prevention have yet been verified through clinical trials on humans.

I am probably healthier for adhering to these dietary modifications for prostate cancer prevention than I would be with my normal eating habits. A low fat diet has many beneficial features that contribute to overall good health. In addition, I have dropped a few unneeded pounds around the waistline and am finding that my running times have dropped slightly.

20

External Beam Radiation

When my PSA went up to 0.4 ng/ml in February, I decided that it was time to move forward with more aggressive treatment. I had tried nutritional therapy for a very short period of time. Really, I had not given it enough time to thoroughly test the concept. However, I knew that I had an aggressive cancer with a Gleason score of 8 and that my PSA had essentially doubled in 4 months. Even though my urologist told me that doubling times were inaccurate at such low PSA levels, I didn't want to lose my window of opportunity for a complete cure. I decided to go ahead with the radiation therapy, reasoning that if the radiation were to be successful, the lower my PSA was when the therapy was undertaken, the better would my chances be for it to be effective.

During the radiation procedure which consists of 38 treatments over 7 ½ weeks, a cubic area of tissue 8cm x 8cm x 8cm is irradiated with 18 million electron volts of photons from a linear accelerator directed at the target area from above, below and from each side as the patient lies on their back on a flat table. X-ray technicians watch the dosage on a screen outside the room where the patient lies and when the required dosage is reached, of 180–200 rads per day, after about 30 seconds, they turn off the x-ray machine. The irradiated area is the "prostate bed" or the site where the prostate tissue was cut out during radical prostatectomy, the bladder neck and the front wall of the rectum. The entire treatment process was painless and required about 10 minutes of my time. I stopped by for my "daily fix" each morning on my way to work, having my morning cup of coffee in the waiting room.

The side effects of external beam radiation had been carefully explained to Beth and me at the time of my initial consultation with Dr. Abraham.

There is the possibility of rectal bleeding six to 12 months after treatment or a change in bowel habits since the rectum is part of the area irradiated. Looseness of the bowel, or more frequent movements may occur and the patient may always have some slight bowel problem. Urinary problems such as painful or more frequent urination may arise after two or three weeks of therapy and last a month or two, although 95 percent of men do not have long lasting incontinence. A further problem may be fatigue which may set in after three to four weeks of radiation therapy and continue until two months after therapy. Finally, the radiation produces increased impotence due to nerve damage. I was told I would need to use Viagra if I did not need it before the therapy and if I did need it before, then afterwards I would need it more often. Or, I may not have any erections at all following the 38 treatments, although sexual drive is not affected. None of this was very encouraging, although my prospects for a complete cure were said to be around 60 percent if no cancer had been found in the lymph nodes or seminal vesicles. There was no need to discontinue my running during treatment or cut back on normal work activities unless I felt it necessary to do so.

It was explained to us that the radiation protocol of 38 treatments had been empirically worked out over decades of research on thousands of patients so that it was just enough to kill cancer cells, but not enough to produce unacceptable levels of tissue or organ damage. The protocol can be interrupted for one or two days as mine was on weekends when I received no treatment, or even for as long as a week, without having an adverse effect on the efficacy. However, the radiation treatment may not be repeated again since it has been shown that cells irradiated have "a memory" which makes them increasingly susceptible to damage if they were to receive a second round of treatment. Thus, anything beyond the 38 treatments could produce serious internal effects. When the "prostate bed" is irradiated, healthy cells as well as cancerous cells are damaged, but the healthy tissue recovers faster, so that over time, the net result is death and elimination of the cancer.

My first visit following the initial consultation was for determining the position of my internal organs prior to commencing with the radiation treatments. In this procedure, I was given barium sulfate via the rectum and bowel and urethra so that the locations of bowel and bladder could be marked externally and used as guides for adjusting the x-ray beam. A tube inserted into the urethra for this purpose instructed in the art of forced levitation which in my case was accompanied by a loud yell. A blood sample for initial PSA testing was taken which later was evaluated at 0.4 ng/ml. It is interesting and worth noting that throughout the 7 ½ weeks of treatment and continuing into the recovery phase, I had PSA testing at both my urologist's and radiation oncologist's laboratories and they were not always the same, although they never differed by more than 0.1 ng/ml. When more than one blood sample is taken from a patient and separate tests run at different labs, they can differ appreciably (by as much as 23 percent) according to the standard used to evaluate the level of PSA (Catalona, 2005).

After being told of the potential side effects from radiation, I decided to use positive affirmations to counteract the negativity. Specific affirmations were, "Everyday in every way I am becoming healthier and healthier and healthier."

"My immune system is strong and getting stronger. It is fully capable of overcoming any disease, cancer or pathogen that may enter my body."

"Cancerous areas are being replaced with healthy, normal cells and tissues."

"I expect the best and with God's help I will attain the best."

At the time of beginning radiation treatment I had been on nutritional therapy for over a month. On the fourth day of treatment I brought up the topic of my nutritional regimen and, surprisingly, Dr. Abraham told me to suspend it immediately. It seems that the vitamins C and E and selenium contain antioxidants that can protect cells, thus reversing the effects of the radiation. Laboratory studies indicate that adding vitamin C to irradiated cells counteracts the cell damage that normally occurs. My having taken these supplements for four out of the 38 days should not be a problem, however, he related, because the 38 days is a long duration treatment anyway. I have to question why I was not informed of the interaction of radiation with nutritional supplements at the very beginning of treatment.

Had I not brought up the topic, I could very well have continued through much of my radiation with neither my doctor nor I realizing that its purpose was being compromised. On the same subject, I have to question why prostate cancer patients are not put on nutritional therapy immediately upon diagnosis of the disease or following initial treatment. In my case, having gone for 5 ½ years between surgery and recurrence, would not this period have possibly been lengthened with the use of the dietary changes advocated by Dr. Charles Myers? Since recurrence following radical prostatectomy occurs in 20–30 percent of men by 5 years and 30–50 percent by 10 years (Catalona and Smith, 1994, Pound et al., 1997, Zincke et al., 1994), does it not make sense to lengthen the post-surgery period without recurrence for up to 50 percent of men? Dietary change and nutritional supplements have the potential to do just this, even though our present knowledge of dosage and effects is rudimentary, and much research is needed in this area. With hindsight and the awareness that I am healthier on a low fat diet lacking red meat supplemented with plant protein, I would have gone on the diet and begun nutritional therapy earlier, immediately post-surgery, had I known of it. For many men, delaying the onset of symptoms following surgery and recurrence is a reality and dietary change with nutritional therapy has the potential to ultimately lengthen lifetimes. Put in practical terms, isn't it a better than equal tradeoff to spend years on a healthy diet taking nutritional supplements if you are able to stick around to enjoy your grandchildren for a longer time and die of other causes instead of advanced metastatic prostate cancer?

21

An Anomalous Result

The 38 radiation treatments progressed as planned with further PSA testing after the 28th and 38th treatment to assess results. As Dr. Abraham explained, my PSA at the 28th treatment should ideally show a drop which would indicate that the cancer was being targeted by the X-rays. However, if the cancer was outside of the radiation area, then the PSA level would not be affected. Yet, there could be no immediate change in PSA and the cancer could still be targeted, but wouldn't fall off until nearer to the 38th treatment. My PSA level after 28 treatments was 0.7 ng/ml, up from the 0.4 ng/ml at the beginning of treatment.

At this point, my radiation oncologist suspended further treatment. His reasoning was that the radiation was not targeting the cancer and we should not continue with the remainder of the treatments as I would only incur unnecessary side effects from radiation exposure. He instructed me to return to the nutritional therapy and in a week I would provide another blood sample, have it tested for PSA, and he and I would decide what to do next. Nine out of ten of his patients have a 30 percent drop in PSA after 28 treatments. My urologist came at this turn of events from a different position, however.

Nine days prior to the 0.7 PSA test, Dr. Stonehouse's lab had tested my blood's PSA at 0.4 ng/ml. He was of the view that the 0.7 ng/ml was due to an erroneous test result. He had never seen a PSA level rise as much as mine had (0.4 to 0.7 in five weeks) and felt it unwise to base treatment decisions on only one PSA test. His lab's results indicated that my PSA had been essentially constant over the period of nutritional and radiation therapies. Dr. Stonehouse was of the view that the radiation therapy should not have been discontinued and that it should resume immediately to complete the program. The 38 treatments were, in his view, my last opportunity to achieve a complete cure and that ought not to be compromised on the basis of one "erroneous PSA reading."

In addition, Dr. Stonehouse offered an alternative explanation for my elevated PSA if we assumed the test result to be accurate. His explanation was based on the fact that when the prostate gland is irradiated it produces an excess amount of PSA, so why shouldn't prostate cancer cells do the same? Because of this, an increase in PSA following radiation treatment is not unexpected. In fact, Dr. Abraham had seen slight PSA elevation before in several patients at 28 days of treatment. Later, these patients' PSA levels dropped.

The week between my radiation oncologist's PSA tests came and went. My second PSA test was 0.6 ng/ml, a drop from 0.7 over the one week period. We discussed this latest test result and decided that I should go back onto the radiation therapy to complete the 38 treatments and off the nutritional therapy. He reiterated my urologist's explanation that prostate cancer cells "leak" PSA upon radiation and so the PSA level in the blood rises. The 0.7 PSA level had apparently not been erroneous, but indicative of PSA "leakage." He was not worried about the interruption of treatments interfering with overall effectiveness of the protocol. Furthermore, he did not really know what my test results meant. I later asked Dr. Stonehouse if my high Gleason score of 8 could predispose cancer cells to greater leakage upon irradiation. He replied that when the Gleason score is high, as 9 or 10, the PSA given off becomes much less.

As I neared the end of the 38 treatments, I had experienced little in the way of side effects. There had been some increased frequency of urination and some increased flatulence at times, but little more. "No pain, no gain" does not apply, I was told and my minimal side effects did not equate with any lack of effectiveness of the radiation in killing the cancer cells. Towards the end of the treatments, in addition to the above, I experienced some mild burning sensation upon urinating. Diarrhea was never a problem, nor constipation. Nor was fatigue any more of a problem than usual. Neither can I say that my sexual potency was negatively affected. In short, I can honestly say that few if any of the predicted side effects ever came to fruition, and my continence, bowel behavior and potency are as good today as they were before the radiation therapy. Any side effects that occurred during the 38 days did not persist afterwards. My radiation oncologist told me I was an exception—that most men after surgery and radiation do not have any continence or potency left.

22

Enter the Medical Oncologist

I had continued running throughout the 8½ weeks it took to complete the 38 radiation treatments. I never felt that my energy level was at all reduced by the treatments, nor was the intensity of my training any different than normal. In fact, I ran a 66.5 second 400 meter race indoors on the 28th day of treatment, for me a very good time.

At the end of the 38th treatment, a blood sample was taken, evaluated and returned a test result of PSA = 0.5 ng/ml, a further drop over the 0.6 at 28 days + one week, thus confirming the existence of a "spike" in PSA during the latter phase of radiation treatment. If true, then the X-ray beam had to have been targeting cancer cells, a very encouraging result and the hoped for outcome of the therapy. One month later, my PSA had fallen to 0.2 ng/ml. At this point I was advised to resume nutritional therapy.

After completing the radiation therapy the usual trend is that the PSA level drops to a nadir, then it may stay there or go back up if the cancer is still present. Six to 12 or sometimes 12–18 months are required to establish a nadir. My PSA levels dropped to a nadir of <0.1 ng/ml at 7–10 months following treatment. Then, they started to increase. At about this time, my radiation oncologist moved to a new position in Boston and since my radiation therapy was complete, I returned to Dr. Stonehouse for medical attention related to my condition. My PSA rose to 0.2 ng/ml in July, 2003 and to 0.4 ng/ml in September. In my urologist's words, "Your cancer has metastasized." In his view, the rise following a nadir meant that a few cells, somewhere outside of the prostate bed, had escaped radiation treatment and now were beginning to grow and multiply. The cells could be anywhere in my body and until my PSA reached 2 or 3 it was not possible to locate them. At a PSA of 2 or 3 they might be found with a prostascint scan, but until that time, there was little to do but watchful waiting and monitoring of the PSA.

When my PSA rose to 0.2 ng/ml, I was referred to a local medical oncologist, Dr. William L. Stanley, whom Beth and I went to visit in early August, 2003. His recommendation was to continue PSA testing until a trend was established. However, in early stages of cancer growth there is little that is recommended as a treatment beyond the nutritional therapy I was already doing. Dr. Stanley recommended taking soy protein on a daily basis. Available in powder form, it may be blended with fruit juice and solid fruit to make a delicious shake. I added 30 grams of this a day to my nutritional regimen.

Dr. Stanley is a believer in holistic medicine and feels it has value in treating cancer, especially for someone like myself with low PSA, but with "metastatic disease." I related to him my use of positive affirmations, prayer and that I was a long time practitioner of transcendental meditation. He believes in the power of the mind to bring about healing, but appreciates the fact that we don't as yet have an understanding of how to focus the mind properly to control the healing process.

My visits to Dr. Stanley continued and my PSA crept up slowly. In April, 2004 with a PSA = 0.8 ng/ml, it was suggested I have a bone scan and CAT scan. These came back negative. Sometimes, I was told, as a tumor grows it produces correspondingly smaller amounts of PSA. In a very small number of men a sizeable tumor is detectable even though the PSA level is low. The scans, for me merely precautionary in this sense, served another purpose, however. They provided a baseline of visual information that later, if necessary, could be used for comparative purposes should my disease progress to an advanced stage.

23

My Training Regimen

The summer of 2003 was very successful for me as a runner. In June at the Empire State Senior Games I had run a hand-timed 13.72 for 100 meters, a 29.3 for 200 meters and 66.4 for 400 meters. The 100 meter time was the best I had run at that distance since prior to my surgery in 1996. Following the Senior Games, I was able to continue training with little interruption through the rest of June and July, and was feeling optimistic about my preparation for participating in the Empire State Games in Buffalo, New York on July 25.

My training program for the Games consisted of one day of weight training emphasizing both upper and lower body lifts, one day of a distance run of not more than 2 miles, one day of sprint training, and one day of cross training in a swimming pool. My workouts build upper body as well as lower body strength, essential for sprinters, and I used a distance run and interval training on the track and in the pool to build anaerobic capacity. As the Games neared, I replaced the swimming workout with another day of sprint training. I provide time for recovery between daily workouts whether they are in the pool, on the track or in the weight room. Often I allow for a day off between hard workouts so that a typical week might find me training four days a week and resting for three, or if I feel like it, training five days a week and resting two. By this regimen, I try to avoid overtraining, making sure that my workouts are difficult, but psychologically enjoyable. I save my hardest runs for competition, but work up close to that point in my daily training so as not to bring fatigue to the actual race. Note that this was not how I approached training and competition when I was younger. As a masters runner in my 30's and 40's, I recovered faster from hard workouts and could train harder than I can now. I try to listen to the message my body is sending me—am I feeling fresh and ready to go each day or listless on the track with legs that feel like they have weights attached?

I use a Hatha yoga routine twice a week to build flexibility and use butt kicks and high knee skipping on the track and in place to promote strength over the entire range of motion essential to sprinting. Rapid arm pumps that simulate the sprinting motion while sitting on the ground are useful for strengthening the upper body and preparing it for the integrated motion of fast running. I warm up before workouts on the track by jogging a quarter mile, then stretching, then a half mile of running the straightaways and jogging the curves, working up to near full speed on the straightaways. Similarly, I warm down after my workout by jogging at least a quarter mile or its equivalent in the swimming pool.

The day of the Games arrived, but the skies were overcast and there was a strong headwind coming up the straightaway to slow down runners. As a result, my times in the 100 and 200 meter races were slow—14.38 for 100m and 30.00 for 200 m. In the 400 meters, however, I finished in an electronically timed 65.98 seconds in spite of the headwind at the end of the race. I took the gold medal for age 60–64 in the 400m and silver medals in the 100m and 200m. I later learned that my 400m time placed me 22nd in the U.S. in my 60–64 age group for that distance according to the 2003 outdoor Masters Track & Field Rankings (Clingan and Patz, 2004).

A 400 meter race is an endeavor that I have grown better at over the years in the sense that it was once something, as a high school runner, that I dreaded. I have gotten used to the pain of the last 100 meters of the race or perhaps my pain threshold has increased. I now enjoy the distance, but I think also that I now know how to train for it such that the race no longer represents such a formidable challenge. To run 400 meters, one has to run fast and be relaxed doing it. This means that good form is essential in order not to waste energy through inefficient motion. It also requires good upper and lower body strength. I have used repeat 300's in order to build speed and then, 500 or 600 meter repeats in order to build endurance. I used to use starting blocks when I was running under 60 seconds. Now, I do not, feeling that the advantage gained is minimal. I try to run the first 200 meters a second or two faster than the last 200. Relaxing on the back stretch is essential. I have always run curves well. In the 400, relaxing on the curve comes easy to me, so that when I come off the final curve at 300 meters, I try to concentrate on vigorous arm motion to carry my form. Otherwise, my legs do not sustain my speed and my form falls apart. The last 100 meters is always painful, but with proper training, the pain is minimized and tolerated better.

Based on my 200 meter race time of 29.3 seconds run in 2003 at age 60, I refigured my percent increase in 200 meter time over the intervening period since 1996 when I had run 27.3 seconds for the distance. My times had declined at the rate of 1.05 percent per year, a rate of decline greater than the 0.42 percent per year between the ages of 39 and 53, but still considerably better than the loss of two percent a year in physical vitality for a sedentary person that Dr. Walter Bortz predicts (Bortz, 1996). When I figured the rate of decline overall between ages 39 and 60, my 200 meter time had increased at the rate of 0.65 percent per year, still close to the half a percent per year that Bortz said should characterize a fit person who maintains an active lifestyle and is between the ages of 30 and 70. Dr. Bortz says that "the strength and benefit of exercise are now without serious challenge. It's the strongest medicine there is. But knowing that on a rational basis and translating it into a daily activity is the tough part." This is why an organization like the Syracuse Chargers Track Club that provides some kind of running activity for all levels of abilities and interests and for all ages is so beneficial to a community.

24

Good Health Finds Its Home

It had been eight years since my initial diagnosis of prostate cancer and a radical prostatectomy which Beth and I and my urologist had hoped would produce a cure. For five and a half years we had thought that the cancer was gone, all removed with the rest of the prostate in the surgery. Then, when the PSA tests revealed the cancer was still present, there had been a series of 38 radiation treatments designed to kill any cancer cells still present in the "prostate bed." The cancer was still there, however, and now my PSA was slowly increasing again. Statistics show that I am not alone. Many men have had prostatectomies followed by radiation without producing a cure. In the words of Dr. Susan Slovin of Memorial Sloan-Kettering Cancer Center, I am experiencing "biochemical relapse," locally advanced prostate cancer which shows no disease on a bone scan or CAT scan, but is associated with a rising PSA.

Throughout the past nine years I have continued to train and run competitively and successfully. Outside of my recovery period from the prostatectomy there has been little or no downtime related to the presence of the cancer. Nor have I experienced any complications or lingering problems related to either the surgery or radiation treatments that have in any way affected my running. I am able to train as hard today as ever and my body responds with a high level of fitness and physical health and well being. In fact, although I cannot prove it, my level of health and fitness has probably been a positive factor in my ability to recover from cancer treatments. An improved physical resiliency, cultivated through regular physical conditioning, has seemed to underlie my response to medical treatment.

If I could clone myself and give one being a running regimen and the other a sedentary lifestyle, then observe the effects of prostate cancer and its treatment on both beings, I could definitively answer the question as to whether running is a beneficial factor in overcoming or coping with prostate cancer, but I cannot. It is thus my hypothesis that runners are better able to cope with prostate cancer and its progression than non-runners. Certainly, running bolsters the immune system and has a myriad of additional benefits for both physical and mental health. To test my hypothesis would be difficult, however, since groups of runners and non-runners selected randomly would not differ just in presence or absence of running, but would have quite different pre-test histories, confounding factors that would complicate interpretations of test results. Perhaps someday someone will attempt to set up such an experiment, but so far it has not been done. We are left with inference and supposition and clues resulting from pieces of the puzzle that only form part of a picture.

The Lance Armstrong Foundation is testing men with prostate cancer in an intensive exercise program which, at best, will show that men with cancer can benefit physically from an exercise program. What it will not do is indicate whether exercise has therapeutic value, i.e., whether lifting weights, running, swimming or cycling can arrest or slow down the progression of cancer. It may very well have such an effect, but their testing procedures are not designed to conclusively show such value. Nevertheless, the Foundation's efforts represent a positive step forward in understanding and demonstrating the benefits of exercise in older men and their work will provide basis for their fight against testicular cancer. Recently, a study of 8 to 12 sixty-year-old men that had been in a vigorous exercise program for 14 years indicated that a low fat diet and/or strenuous exercise resulted in changes in blood serum hormones and growth factors relative to a control group of sedentary men. When the serum from the active men was added to prostate cancer cells in vitro, tumor cell growth was reduced and apoptosis (programmed cell death) of tumor cells increased (Barnard et al., 2003).

Lance Armstrong, in his book "It's Not About the Bike: My Journey Back to Life," reports on the chances he was given to survive testicular cancer (Armstrong, 2001). Following his successful treatment, he asked his oncologist in retrospect what he believed his chances of full recovery to have been. His doctor replied, "probably less than three percent." Yet, Lance was able to not only survive his cancer, but go on to win seven consecutive races of the Tour de France. When initially diagnosed, his cancer had metastasized to the brain. When surgery to remove the tumors was performed, doctors found, remarkably, that the tumors were necrotic. Did Lance's high level of fitness have anything to do with the tumors being made up of dead tissue? I can only speculate that perhaps it did. Certainly, his fitness was a factor in how his body was able to tolerate the chemotherapy. The Foundation believes that knowledge is power and urges cancer survivors to "live strong", i.e., to become informed and involved in the shared decision-making of their cancer experience. What this means is to read up on your disease so that you understand it and what the possible cures are. Then, you can discuss your disease intelligently with your doctor and make the best decisions regarding treatment options. The more informed and empowered patient has a better chance at long-term survival.

While he was in the hospital, Lance Armstrong made up an acronym out of the word, C-A-N-C-E-R: C—Courage, A—Attitude, N—Never give up, C—Curability, E—Enlightenment, R—Remembrance of fellow patients. Lance redefines cancer not as a form of death, but as a part of life. Having courage in the face of death and a positive attitude that includes acquiring knowledge and never giving up produces an enlightened mind and a belief in the curability of the cancer. Survivors have something to pass along to those who are recently diagnosed. When we remember others who suffer and reach out to them in support, we transform ourselves from persons dying of a disease to persons who choose to live regardless of the outcome. In essence, we create the conditions necessary for survival by our attitude towards our own mortality. Where the proper conditions for life are present, good health finds its home.

25

Masters Runners—Their Stories

If there is a constant in cases of prostate cancer or any illness, it is that everyone's physical or medical situation is somewhat unique, different in one or more ways from another person's. This fact must be what doctors find fascinating and challenging about their work and, of course at times, difficult. There is always a need to consider the individual's specifics of age, medical history, disease symptoms, as well as to know of the recent medical advances in the treatment of prostate cancer.

As I talked with other masters runners who, like myself, had been diagnosed with prostate cancer, I began to realize that each person had his own story to tell. Some were young when they discovered their disease; some were older and beyond the point where surgery was a possibility. Some opted for radiation as a treatment; others opted for prostatectomies; others for "watchful waiting". In order to illustrate the range of circumstances that masters athletes may find themselves in when diagnosed with cancer, and to provide an example of how very different each person's experience with prostate cancer may be, I interviewed four masters runners. The runners ranged in age from 60 to 77 when first diagnosed. They ranged in ability as athletes. One had been a national champion triple jumper and hurdler; two were sprinters, another a distance runner, and one competed in road races as well as short distance events. I have tried to include some of their post-operative histories of recuperation as runners. One underwent surgery for removal of the prostate, another elected radiation treatment and two have employed "watchful waiting". All returned to active competition following either surgery, radiation treatment or during their "watchful waiting". Here are their stories.

Howard C. MacMillan
Liverpool, New York
(presently of Brick, New Jersey)

Howard started running in 1967 at age 42 after being inspired by Kenneth H. Cooper's book, <u>The New Aerobics</u>. He entered his first 5K road race, the Unity Life Road Race, 11 years later and placed second in the 50–59 age group. His performance inspired Howard to try something more challenging, whereupon at age 53, he joined the Syracuse Chargers Track Club and started running in local Chargers-sponsored track meets.

Since that first meet, Howard excelled in the sprints, taking first place in the 400 meters at age 70 in the U.S. National Masters Indoor Championships in 72.54 seconds and second place in the 60 meter dash in 9.05 seconds. Howard's efforts on the track have produced 17 first places at Eastern Regional meets and 55 first places at Empire State Games competitions.

Howard holds numerous Chargers Track Club records from the 50's age group on up as well as having been part of relay teams that set records at the Empire State Games in the 4x100m (age 70–79) and 4x400m (age 60–69). He held the Empire State Games record for age 70–74 in the 400 meters at 72.1 seconds and currently holds the Eastern Regionals record in the 200 meters at 28.4 seconds for the 70–74 age group.

Although his best races were 400 meters and shorter, Howard regularly participated in road races through age 76. His training regimen included lifting weights, speed work on the track and longer endurance runs on the roads. At age 74, his summer, 2000 track meets included the Empire State Senior Games and the Empire State Games. In 2002, Howard received the New Jersey USA Track & Field 70–79 year old "sprinter of the year" award.

Since 2002, Howard has not actively competed on a regular basis in track & field, although in 2006 he entered and won the 100 meters in the 80–84 age group in the New Jersey Senior Olympics. In 2001, he had arthroscopic surgery for a torn medial meniscus of the left knee. Two surgeries have resulted in arthritis developing and now the left knee is larger than the right and the stride in that leg is shorter than the right. His times on the track and road were suffering, yet a stress test showed his maximum heart rate to be 178 beats per minute. In his doctor's words, "You have the heart of a young man." Howard walks about 4 miles, rides a bike 3 miles (except in winter), does 32 pushups and 20 minutes of stretching and other exercises each day to maintain his fitness.

In July, 1998 at age 72, Howard was diagnosed with prostate cancer following a biopsy in which a small focus of adenocarcinoma was found in the left side of his prostate. The cancer showed up in one out of four sample cores. The biopsy was recommended by his family doctor following a slight rise in his PSA scores: 0.77 (March, 1993), 0.83 (April, 1995), 1.02 (April, 1997), 1.04 (July, 1998). Howard's cancer graded out to a Gleason score of 6 and was categorized at T2A. His PSA score had risen to 1.41 in December, 1998. The following blood test sample was sent to a different laboratory than previous tests. Further PSA scores from the new lab were: 0.9 (April, 1999), 1.0 (July, 1999), 0.9 (October, 1999), 1.0 (January, 2000), 0.7 (April, 2000), 0.9 (July, 2000). In November, 2000, Howard's urologist had his blood samples sent back to the original lab which had done his PSA analysis through December, 1998. His PSA level came back as 1.3, the same as it had been previously, but 0.4 ng/ml higher than the second lab had last determined it to be. A second PSA test done at the same time by a different, but equivalent procedure, yielded a value of 1.8 ng/ml. Either Howard's PSA level had dropped, then risen again by a half unit or laboratory B's procedures were different enough to make their PSA determinations lower by a half unit than those of laboratory A. In 2001, Howard moved to New Jersey and another lab did his PSA analyses. These were 1.63 (April, 2002), 1.93 (January, 2003), 1.42 (January, 2004), and 2.01 (September, 2004). In 2006, his PSA was 2.29 which since then has risen modestly, but Howard continues to monitor his cancer with twice yearly PSA tests.

There is no reason to believe that all laboratories that do PSA analyses should independently come up with identical test results. There is a measure of error involved in any laboratory testing procedure. Statistically, there is an "error variance" associated with PSA testing. I am fairly sure that doctors know what that degree of error is, but may not tell patients.

In Howard's testing, it is most likely the case that his PSA levels changed not because of any change in his cancer, but because a different lab did the analysis. The error variance of repeated tests run between labs is probably greater than that of repeated tests run by the same lab and this would explain Howard's test results.

Howard's PSA scores have been low for a male in his 70's, so he has taken a "watchful waiting" approach to treatment. He realized that as he grew older he was losing the window of opportunity on surgery, should that course of action ever prove necessary. His urologist did not like to do surgery on males over 70, but characterized Howard as "a good bet for surgery" due to his history as a masters athlete even though at the time, Howard was in his mid-70's. Surgery was still an option, therefore, but due to the low magnitude of his PSA, and the fact that it was not clearly rising, Howard did not elect surgery.

Howard's urologist recommended dietary supplements along with the "watchful waiting." These have included vitamin E (500 mg/day; Howard takes a 400 mg capsule and gets an additional 100 mg with a multivitamin.), selenium (200 mcg/day), green tea and soy products all along with a low to moderate fat diet. Several years ago, after reading some cautionary literature about excess vitamin E, he reduced the amount to 50 mg/day.

Through his diagnosis and much of his "watchful waiting", Howard continued to train and compete in track meets and road races. Like many men who have been diagnosed with prostate cancer, he feels no ill effects from his disease. Unlike many men with prostate cancer, however, Howard knows the disease is there and he is watching its presence carefully and regularly through PSA testing.

Robert Metzner
Syracuse, New York

Bob Metzner began his running career as a senior in high school where he ran the half mile and continued it in the army as a sprinter. He had attended Syracuse University at 17 years of age, but didn't graduate until he was 29. His education was interrupted due to service in the Army Air Corps in World War II and later by a bout with tuberculosis which required four years of treatment. In his 50's, Bob was encouraged to stay in shape by guidelines set up by the President's Council on Physical Fitness, but it was not until he was 65 years old that he decided to train for the County Senior Games which were held in Syracuse in 1990. In that meet Bob placed second in the 100 meters with a time of 18.2 which was the beginning of serious competition and was followed with an 8.6 sec indoors in the 55 meter dash. These early successes, however, were followed by a foot injury, apparently arthritis related. After numerous visits to foot specialists and spending two years in physiotherapy, his running career was terminated and Bob moved into field events which placed less stress on his foot. A stationery bicycle and Cybex machines at the YMCA, where Bob goes three times a week, now provide cardiovascular fitness and strength. As a member of the Syracuse Chargers Track Club, he has participated in most of the Empire State Games and Senior Games held in New York since 1989. In the 2004 Empire State Games, in the 75–79 age class, Bob earned gold medals in the javelin, long jump and high jump and a silver medal in the discus. His best marks in that age class in those events were 19.64 m, 2.58 m, 1.02 m and 21.78 m, respectively.

Bob first learned he had prostate cancer in 1985 at age 60 when it was detected during a routine physical. A digital rectal exam found a lump and a consequent biopsy was positive for "a well-differentiated adenocarcinoma" about one centimeter in size. Bob's urologist recommended immediate surgery and Bob learned about treating impotency with penile implants and likely incontinence after surgery. Even though surgery offered the prospect of curing the prostate cancer, these aftereffects discouraged Bob from going ahead with his urologist's recommendation. Bob did not have any inordinate fear of cancer, had had TB and undergone a lengthy convalescence, and had, and still does have, a strong religious faith that God can heal illnesses. Bob went to several Man-to-Man meetings and read up on the disease. His personal physician told Bob that if he was uncomfortable with the surgery, not to go ahead with it, and so Bob elected a "watchful waiting" approach.

Back in 1985, PSA tests did not exist, so it was not until several years later that Bob found out that his PSA tested at 6.8 ng/ml. Thereafter, his

PSA rose to 14 ng/ml during a particularly stressful period, but came back down to 6.8 ng/ml (June, 2001), having dropped for the three years prior. In December, 2004 it was still at 6.8 ng/ml, but by early 2007 had risen suddenly to 30 ng/ml. Bob's urologist put him on Lupron and subsequently, Zoladex which brought his PSA down. Since the initial diagnosis in 1985, Bob has had several bone scans and ultrasounds to follow the progress of the cancer. The Lupron and Zoladex have brought about fatigue, loss of libido and hot flashes, but Bob still manages to get to the YMCA for one hour workouts twice a week. He competed in the Empire State Senior Games this year and earned gold medals in his events even though he was suffering the side effects of the Zoladex. At age 82, the nodule in his prostate appears to be growing and determined treatment is required.

Bob follows the Pritikin diet which is low-fat and he feels that this helped to keep his cancer under control in the early years following diagnosis. He consumes about 10 grams of fat per day, eats low-fat beef and chicken and takes a multiple vitamin daily. Five years after being diagnosed, Bob began to compete in masters track and field which he continues to do today. His "watchful waiting", effective for 21 years, would seem to support his initial decision to reject the surgery. His advice to older males is to keep a positive outlook on life, maintain a proper diet, stay in good physical shape and be knowledgeable enough about your health that you can make your own decisions.

Russell More
Fayetteville, New York

Russell is one of those rare individuals that performs well in sprints and also logs high mileage totals on the roads. His best events are 100m and 200m in which he received All-American status in 1997 at age 76 with times of 16.2 and 35.3 seconds, respectively. Yet, in 1982, Russ logged a total of 1853 miles and ran the New York City Marathon in 3:58:43. Since he resumed running at age 57 and not having run since high school, Russ has averaged 100 miles of running per month. Russell's sprint performances are all the more remarkable since he does not do interval training.

Rather, his sprint training comes at the end of long training runs. In 1996 at age 75, Russell earned 10 gold medals in Empire State Games and New York Senior Games competition, and presently holds several Syracuse Chargers Track Club age 75–79 sprint records.

Russell's PSA tests had been stable at between 2.5–3.7 from 1991–95 when, in 1996, they went up to 4.3, then to 5.2 in 1997. In August, 1998, when his PSA levels were at 4.5, Russell was diagnosed with prostate cancer, staged as T2A (Walsh, 1995) and elected radiation treatment. He first started on hormonal therapy, taking Lupron (leuprolide acetate) shots to cut testosterone production and starve the hormone sensitive cancer cells, reducing the size of his prostate.

Russell's urologist ruled out prostatectomy as a treatment option because Russell was 77 years of age. This was older than 70 years, the age at which his doctor felt surgery was no longer viable as an option due to difficulties with tissues healing properly in older men. Lupron is a chemical that interferes with the normal activity of the hypothalamus in the brain which signals the pituitary gland to produce intermediate chemicals, luteinizing hormone (LH) and follicle-stimulating hormone (FSH), in the testosterone production chain. The pituitary is tricked into ceasing production of LH and FSH, so testosterone supply to the prostate is eventually cut off. By December, his PSA levels had dropped to <0.1 ng/ml. On January 13, 1999, radiation pellets or "seeds" were implanted by computer imaging in Russell's prostate. The implantation required an overnight hospital stay and he was allowed to go home the next day after it became clear that he was able to urinate a fixed volume of fluid. He continued with the Lupron shots until mid-April, and post-implantation PSA levels have remained at < 0.1 ng/ml as tested in April and August, 1999, January and July, 2000, and January, 2001. Russell continued to run up until the day before his implant procedure and his first run after the radiation implant was in eight days when he ran two-and-one-half miles at a 13 minute/mile pace. Another eight days after this he competed as a member of a 4x200m relay team in a local indoor track meet.

Russell has noticed no serious long-term effects of the radiation treatment although he still has "hot flashes". The Lupron reduced his testosterone levels and Russell feels it negatively affected his running temporarily by reducing his sprint speed. For three months following treatment, Russell experienced painful urination. Additionally, a burning sensation which was only supposed to have lasted six weeks, persisted for six months. His continence is fine today.

In May, 2000, Russell spent ten days in the hospital for an abdominal aneurysm, but recovered rapidly. By July, Russell was walking at a twelve minute per mile pace, and by November (age 79) was competing on the track again.

In May, 2001, Russell was in the hospital again. This time it was surgery for a brain aneurysm, but due to his high level of fitness, Russell amazed his doctors who hadn't expected the rapid and high degree of recovery that he exhibited. By fall, he was running and playing golf again, looking expectantly to competing over the winter in track and field events. Russell has participated regularly in the Empire State Games and in the 2004 Empire State Senior Games won 5 medals, one in each event he entered.

On his 83rd birthday in November, 2004 Russell, rose at 4:30 a.m. and ran 5 miles, as he did every day. This time it was 23 seconds faster than on his birthday in 2003. He still runs and competes today at age 85, although his early morning runs have diminished. His PSA remains <0.1.

William R. Townsend
Liverpool, New York

Bill's running career dates back to his college days in the 1940's when he was a hurdler and jumper on the track team at the University of Maryland. Like many of us, Bill was an active runner early in life, then did not run again until much later. He resumed running competitively in the 1980's under the tutelage of Oscar Jensen and before the decade was out had won five national championships in the hurdles, three in the triple jump and two in the long jump. Bill competed in the World Veteran's Games in 1987 in Melbourne, Australia and in 1989 in Eugene, Oregon in the 60–64 year age group, placing 8th in the 100 m hurdles (17.74 sec at Eugene) in both Games and also competing in the long jump, triple jump and 300 m hurdles. In 1991, at the age of 64 (60–64 age group), Bill won five gold medals in the javelin, long and triple jump, 110 m hurdles, and the 4 x 100 m relay in the Empire State Games held in Albany, New York. He also took a silver medal in the 100 m dash. His most memorable performance, however, was setting the Canadian 100 m hurdles record of 17.98 sec for the 60–64 age group in the 1988 North American Games in Toronto. In the same meet, Bill ran on the gold medal winning United States 4 x 100 m relay team. Bill considers his top performances to have come in the 60–64 age group for which he also holds the Syracuse Chargers Track Club record in the 300 m hurdles. Although Bill Townsend has established his credentials as a masters athlete, he also holds the rank of Master Official in the New York Association of U.S.A. Track & Field. Bill is often recognized as an official at local as well as regional and, occasionally, at national track and field meets at high school, college and masters levels.

It was in January, 1994 that Bill requested a PSA test during a routine physical examination. It came back at 5.4 ng/ml and Bill's urologist found cancer in his prostate, although his bone scan was negative. His urologist explained the various options for treatment and let Bill decide what to do. Bill sought a second opinion and it was to have a retropubic radical prostatectomy, but Bill's educated decision was to go ahead with a perineal radical prostatectomy which he had in March, 1994 at age 68. His surgeon found clear margins and there was no cancer in the lymph nodes. Bill was walking the day after his surgery and spent five days in the hospital. He had not given his own blood prior to surgery, but did begin kegel exercises one-and-one-half months before surgery. His doctor recommended doing over 100 per day; Bill did 300 per day, continued with them after surgery, and still did them several times a week for some time thereafter. Bill used disposable pads for six weeks, but his incontinence soon ceased to be a problem. Following his March surgery, Bill was back officiating at track meets in May and June. He reported few complications following surgery, only a minor bladder infection, and the fact that he discovered he was allergic to the antibiotic, Cipro. He continued to take regular PSA tests to monitor his recovery from surgery. Bill competed in the National Masters

Outdoor Championships in August, 1997 and continued to compete until fall, 1999 at age 72 when he ceased running competitively for reasons unrelated to his prostate surgery. There are simply few competitors in Bill's events in the 70 years and over age groups. Up until the time of this interview in August, 2000, Bill still exercised regularly with a stretching and walking routine and took a mixture of herbs for arthritis.

Bill had this advice for males over 50: take a physical each year and cover "all the bases". Be informed so that you can know all the proper tests you need. Be responsible for your health. Follow a good, nutritious diet and get proper rest. Bill's urologist felt that running had been a positive factor for Bill because of his age at time of surgery. The muscular control that running provided was felt to have facilitated his recovery, leading his doctor to comment that he wished he "had 200 more patients like you".

Unfortunately, Bill is no longer with us, having died of pancreatic cancer several years after I interviewed him, in March, 2003.

All of the runners described above continued to compete regardless of the presence of prostate cancer. Of course, all have taken some measure of control over their cancer, including watchful waiting, and none were in stages of advanced disease where the cancer had metastasized and spread to other organs. Yet, the four cases illustrate the point that each man's cancer is unique and therefore must be treated differently. Howard chose to watch his cancer carefully, and to date this seems to have been a sound choice. He still exercises regularly, but does not compete anymore. Russ continues to run and compete and is a splendid role model for runners in their 80's. Bill is not here now, but his running did not end because of prostate cancer nor did his life. Bob continues his diet, but at 22 years post-diagnosis, has gone from a "watchful waiting" approach to hormone blockade, yet he still competes in field events. His cancer is presently under control.

The decision by these four runners as to type of treatment was not made by following a simple formula written down in a medical journal or popular treatise on prostate cancer. It is something that each man determined for himself based on advice from his doctor, his understanding and interpretation of the disease's progression in his body, his family history and his own personal judgment. All presently have their cancers under control through one means or another (excepting Bill), and if there is any constant in their stories, it is that all employed different treatment protocols.

26

Advances in Treatment

I consider myself extremely fortunate to have discovered my cancer at an early stage. I could just as easily be a walking "time bomb", waiting for some symptom of cancer to appear that would drive me to the doctor to seek relief. The odds, then, would not be in my favor for a complete cure. As it was, my cancer was caught early when the prospects for a cure were high. Prostate cancer victims whose disease has progressed to an advanced stage before it is detected often die an early and painful death. Francois Mitterand, Timothy Leary, Floyd Patterson, Jerry Orbach, Linus Pauling, and Eldridge Cleaver are familiar names of men who are no longer with us, but who could still be alive had their cancers been detected early.

My son will need to start taking yearly PSA tests or their equivalent when he is 40 years old because his father and brother-in-law both had prostate cancer at an early age and there is a heritable component to the disease. Why did I develop prostate cancer? What caused it? To my knowledge it is not in my family, but then I may have family members who died of it before medical tests for the disease's detection were available and their deaths were attributed to other factors. Medical researchers at Mount Sinai School of Medicine in New York City have found mutated versions of the gene, KLF6, in many prostate tumors which disrupt KLF6's normal role of inhibiting cell growth (Narla et al., 2001; 2005). At some point, when a genetic test for prostate cancer becomes available, I will be tested, and so will my son. Still, it does not mean that my cancer was inherited even if I test positive for an altered prostate cancer gene. All that is inherited is the predisposition. The cancer could still have been related to some predominant factor or factors in my environment. We all live in a world full of known and unknown carcinogens arising from man-made pollutants present in water, soil and air. Not enough is presently known about the origins of the disease, however, to answer questions related to cause.

The best that men, especially middle-aged, can presently do is to recognize the importance of early diagnosis of prostate cancer and begin to have the simple PSA blood test conducted yearly by family physicians and at an early age, 50 years according to the American Cancer Society (2004), earlier at age 40 if in a high-risk group such as African-American or those whose brothers or fathers have had prostate cancer. Prostate cancer is more common in African-Americans than in other ethnic/racial groups. The PSA test, developed by Dr. William J. Catalona in 1991, has since played a major role in early diagnosis and treatment of prostate cancer and has contributed to increased rates of survival for men with the disease (Catalona et al., 1991). Now, with PSA testing, cancers can be detected 5 to 13 years sooner than they would be without the screening test, often when the cancer is confined to the prostate gland.

Diet appears to be a predisposing factor in the incidence of prostate cancer just as it is with other cancers. The American Cancer Society recommends a low-fat, high-fiber diet rich in vegetables, fruit and soy as effective in reducing one's chances of developing prostate cancer. Using the Harvard Alumni group again, Ralph Paffenbarger (Sesso et al.,2001) studied the effects of specific types of alcohol consumption and the risk of prostate cancer. Seven thousand six hundred and twelve men of an average age of 66.6 years were followed between 1988 and 1993 and using previous records from 1977 and during college. Three hundred sixty-six developed prostate cancer. Results indicated that wine or beer consumption was unassociated with prostate cancer, but that moderate liquor consumption increased the risk of prostate cancer by 61–67 percent. Men who began alcohol consumption between 1977 and 1988 doubled their risk of prostate cancer compared to other men who had nearly none or no alcohol consumption during that period. The authors of this study point out, however, that many other studies on alcohol use and prostate cancer risk have been inconclusive.

All men and women should assume as much responsibility for their own health as they are able to. By this I mean becoming familiar with potential health problems they may have or particular predispositions so that one can talk intelligently to their doctor and be given the proper diagnostic tests. In the case of prostate cancer, this is crucial. My doctor did not recommend the PSA test for his male patients. Had I not known about the test and requested it, I would likely today be either unaware of the growing cancer within me or it would have by now spread beyond the prostate and produced symptoms. The digital rectal exam will identify only about 20 percent of prostate cancers. Don't rely on your doctor to be God; he or she is only human. You have a mind and a brain to think with—use them to educate yourself in the ways and necessities of your own health maintenance. Although doctors are trained to do what they do and usually are correct, they do have opinions when a practice or procedure is at all controversial. An opinion on some topic may not be entirely accurate simply because research has not as yet produced a uniform point of view. Your doctor's opinion when it comes to a new diagnostic test or controversial practice may not be the right one for you. You are better off to become as knowledgeable as possible so that you recognize what is controversial and what is not. Only going to see the doctor when problems develop is not taking charge of your own health. The reason for this is that many diseases or health problems that may be treated properly or prevented depend upon early diagnosis. In many cases, the window of opportunity for effective treatment may have passed when the tumor is discovered or when the heart attack arrives. Prostate cancer is in this category.

I have to ask myself why it was that my doctor, Peter Grendle, like others I have since learned, did not recommend the PSA test for his male patients. His initial response, "… there are false positives and false negatives often associated with the test," suggested a more pervasive problem.

Managed care health plans, under which many Americans are insured, have come to emphasize standardization of practice and elimination of unnecessary tests and procedures in the interests of containing health care costs. They are run like a business, so that investors make a profit which, unfortunately for the patient, has become their prime objective rather than patient health. Many medical decisions have thus been taken out of the hands of physicians and other health care personnel. Rather, it is the accountants and businessmen that work for the health care companies that make the decisions. In this light, PSA tests and cancer biopsies that may ultimately prove unnecessary are not cost effective. The person who gets cheated is the one who, like myself, has prostate cancer, but is never tested because PSA tests may not be deemed cost effective. Another person may get tested and have an out-of-range PSA reading, and then receive a negative biopsy, but actually does have cancer (false negative) yet it is dismissed as an age-related increase in PSA—case closed. A second biopsy may have revealed the presence of cancer, but was not cost effective. To what degree are physicians influenced in their medical diagnoses and recommendations by the financially-based procedures of health care companies? The answer is that they are influenced in both overt and subtle ways, and the patient, out of ignorance, is not always in a position to know when their health care is being compromised.

Dr. Stonehouse, my urologist, now tells me that bone scans are not given anymore following a positive biopsy when the PSA level is less than 10 and sometimes even when it is less than 14, depending on the doctor. The reason is that for these patients, only a very low percentage will have cancer outside of the prostate. Bone scans are expensive and insurance companies don't want to pay for them when the chances of a positive scan are small. Yet, in a few cases, there will be patients who need a bone scan for accurate diagnosis of the spread of their prostate cancer, and early treatment, but will not receive one. Of course, money will be saved and that is a guiding principle.

Better diagnostic testing for the disease is emerging from recent research. The "free PSA" test is such an advance (Partin et al., 1996). It is a blood test designed to test for a particular kind of prostate-specific antigen associated with cancer. A high total PSA reading between four and ten may not indicate cancer, only other prostate problems such as age-related enlargement or inflammation. "Free PSA" level is more directly related to cancer. For men whose total PSA is between 4 and 10 ng/ml and have no physical evidence of a tumor, a free PSA less than 25 percent, or even better, less than 10 percent, combined with a biopsy will detect 95 percent of cancers. Since ¾ of men with PSA levels between 4 and 10 ng/ml do not have cancer (American Prostate Society, 1997), the free PSA test can indicate which of those in that PSA range need a biopsy, eliminating 29 percent of negative biopsies.

It is a good practice to chart one's total PSA level over time to observe changes. If the rate of change increases drastically upwards, then it may be a sign that cancer is present and further diagnostic tests are needed. If the rate of increase is constant, a natural trend in men over 40 as the prostate enlarges, and at a low absolute level, then perhaps nothing is remiss. William Catalona suggests using "PSA velocity", the rate of rise in PSA, as a guide to undergoing a biopsy. When the PSA velocity is greater than 0.75 ng/ml per year, he recommends a full biopsy.

Recent research by Dr. Catalona based on a study of 36,000 men over 12 years has shown that a PSA threshold of 2.5 is preferable to the traditional threshold of 4.0 ng/ml (Punglia et al., 2003). That is, for men whose PSA level is greater than 2.5 ng/ml, a prostate cancer biopsy is recommended. Rather than waiting until the PSA reaches 4.0, an earlier biopsy will detect cancer in a significant number of men at a stage when the cancer is more treatable. Thus, the American Cancer Society now recommends consideration of a biopsy when the PSA is above 2.5.

Other research suggests that prostate removal may still be helpful even if the cancer has spread to the lymph nodes (Ward and Zincke, 2003; Ward et al., 2005). The statistics favoring going ahead and removing the prostate under this circumstance indicate an improved response to later hormonal therapy and better long-term survival rates. This was not the view eleven years ago when my surgery was done, but is now the approach taken by my urologist.

Novel new approaches to fighting prostate cancer focus on the molecular level. A vaccine (Provenge) currently seeking FDA approval involves removing immature immune (dendritic) cells from the blood, mixing them with antigens found only on prostate cancer cells and not on healthy cells, and reinjecting them into the blood stream. The dendritic cells display the cancer antigens to the immune system and stimulate the immune system to mount an attack on the cancer cells that possess the antigen.

Another approach aims to strengthen the immune system by injecting PSMA (prostate specific membrane antigen) DNA into the bloodstream. The PSMA DNA could result in the production of antibodies which recognize prostate cancer cells or white blood cells which fight infection.

Another promising approach uses "smart bombs" which are genetic compounds engineered to go only to the prostate cancer cells and signal the cells to die. Cancer cells have lost the mechanism, common in normal cells, that tells them when to die, called "apoptosis", so that they continue to divide.

For patients with advanced prostate cancer, the chemotherapy drug, docetaxel (Taxotere), offers increased survival compared to conventional chemotherapy and is now the standard of care. The combination of docetaxel with other novel cancer agents is an exciting new area of research.

"Personalized medicine" will come into clinical use someday. It is based on the genetic mutation profile of the individual patient and will indicate how that patient may respond more favorably to certain accepted cancer treatments unlike the current protocol that treats patients based entirely on the type of cancer.

The nature of the prostatectomy itself is now changing. Robotic surgery with the da Vinci method involves inserting a video camera through a small incision into the abdominal cavity through which the surgeon conducts the removal of the prostate, viewing his work on a computer monitor. Robotic arms inserted through other small incisions are controlled by the surgeon, doing the work of cutting the prostate away from the tissue and blood vessels that surround it and rebuilding the urinary tract. Robotic surgery involves a much faster recovery period since less tissue is cut during the operation, but we await a decision on the efficacy of the new approach compared to open radical prostatectomy until enough time has passed and comparative data becomes available.

All of these advances present a great deal of hope for men diagnosed with prostate cancer. It is just as insidious a disease in men as breast cancer is in women, but over the years has not received as much attention nor as many research dollars as the latter. As a result, many men are unaware of the facts concerning prostate cancer and the importance of early detection and treatment. I take advantage of every opportunity to relate my experiences to others, both men and women.

27

Take Charge of Your Health

As a runner, I had good health in my favor, which made my surgery and recovery easier and my return to good health faster than if I had not been in top physical condition. Because I discovered my cancer early when I was young at age 53, my recovery was faster than if I had been older. I experienced none of the post-surgery complications that other popular authors of works on prostate cancer have written about such as blood clots, bladder spasms, internal bleeding, and constipation (Korda, 1996; Eisenberg, 1996; Levy, 1999), my hospitalization was of minimal duration with little pain, I was 99 percent continent after 10 weeks and am presently, at age 64, able to continue in competitive sports with no apparent ill effects.

Men recently diagnosed and making their decision as to type of treatment should be aware of a study by Thomas Jang and Justin Bekelman of the Memorial Sloan-Kettering Cancer Center reported at the recent (2007) American Society of Clinical Oncologists meetings where 85,000 men aged 65 and older whose cancer had not yet spread beyond the prostate were evaluated for choice of treatment. The study results indicated that the type of cancer treatment a man gets has a lot to do with the type of specialist he sees first. Urologists recommended surgery 70 percent of the time for men under age 70. Those men who saw both a urologist and a radiation oncologist most often chose radiation over surgery (78 percent). Men over 75 who saw only a urologist were more likely to choose watchful waiting than those men who saw both a urologist and a radiation oncologist. These results make it more essential than ever that men become educated and aware of their options after initial diagnosis so that they can make intelligent decisions. Going to both a urologist and a radiation oncologist to get that "second opinion" makes a good deal of sense.

Becoming educated about prostate cancer and getting a second opinion are what is meant by "taking charge of your health."

There is bias even within the medical profession and often it is not easy for the non-medical person to recognize it. Educated decisions are not made by doctors exclusively; you and I can make wise decisions in association with our urologist or oncologist that are mutual in nature and based in self-education. We may not know as much as a medical doctor, but we can learn the basics of our disease, what the treatments options entail and the advantages and disadvantages of each. We are thus in a better position to distinguish between sound and poor advice or treatments that are controversial when we encounter them.

Transcendental Meditation, Silva Mind Control methods, and prayer arising out of a strong religious faith were useful tools in my coping with cancer and recovery from treatments. Belonging to a community of faith and receiving the prayers of others helped me enormously. I say this without being able to identify exactly the ways or the extent to which these tools were effective. I believe that they all helped just as I believe in the power of God and that we can align ourselves with His or Her power to receive spiritual benefits that not only affect us mentally, but physically as well. Dr. Israel Barken, Chairman of the Prostate Cancer Research and Education Foundation (PC-REF), writes about the M.E.D.S. principles. They are Mental Attitude, Exercise, Diet, Spirituality, and Dr. Barken says we need to take all these "MEDS" on a daily basis. I cannot agree more with him. Finally, I owe much of my well being and favorable recovery from cancer treatments to my wife, Beth, who became nearly as knowledgeable about my disease as I, was compassionate and helpful, and through her innate sense of good humor was an uplifting and stabilizing force, supporting me in untold ways right from the beginning. Our marriage is stronger for having gone through my experience together at every step.

My hope for you, the reader, is that this story may prove enlightening, that it may cause you to take charge of your own health to a greater extent, that it may inform you of some of the facts about prostate cancer and convince you to have regular PSA tests and that it may encourage you to become physically fit, especially if you are middle-aged. If you already have prostate cancer, minimize its psychological impact by making the most of the other qualities of your life and don't let your disease become more important than the normal things you do and enjoy doing each day. Be open about your disease with others because by so doing you overcome your own fears of it and allow the compassion of others to become a healing factor. If you are already a runner, you have chosen to put yourself in the best possible position with regard to your health, knowing that an active lifestyle will be supportive if ever you must face a life-threatening disease.

THE END

Acknowledgements

I wish to thank the following individuals for contributing their personal stories as masters runners and as prostate cancer patients: Howard C. Mac-Millan, Robert Metzner, Russell More, William R. Townsend. For reasons of professional privacy, I have changed the names of my medical practitioners, but am grateful to them for their care of me as a patient and for their reading of and comments on my manuscript. Karl F. Barth, Samuel P. Clemence, Richard A. Ellison, James W. McTarnaghan and Martin Rothenberg reviewed early drafts of this book and contributed encouragement and helpful suggestions. Finally, my wife, Beth M. Drew has been helpful throughout this effort, acting often as a reviewer and providing loving care and advice to me throughout my 11 years as a patient and supportive of my 25 years as a runner, swimmer and cyclist.

Epilogue

Shortly after the 2003 Empire State Games I was involved in a freak biking accident that ended my running career. Riding my road bike in training for an upcoming day trip around one of the finger lakes of upstate New York, I became caught in a sudden rainstorm and ended up on a steep downgrade with poor brakes—a prescription for disaster. As my speed increased uncontrollably on the descent, and I attempted to steer off the highway, I crashed, breaking my right femur at the proximal end which required a partial hip replacement, in medical terms, a hemiarthroplasty. Because of the metal implant which now bears on my hip socket, I am to avoid impact sports such as running which will loosen up the prosthesis and cause me to have a repeat surgical procedure sooner than otherwise. Hip replacements are temporary, and do not last for more than 10 to 20 years, depending upon the individual's health, level of activity, weight, and a number of other factors.

As unfortunate as this was, It was not the prostate cancer that ended my running. In fact, I am still a sprinter in spite of the accident, but in a different sport—masters swimming. I now do my training in a swimming pool instead of at the track. Fifty and 100 meter freestyle are my events of choice; occasionally when my training has gone well I will try a 200 meter freestyle. In the 2004 Empire State Senior Games I placed third in the 100 yard freestyle in 1:20.97 and in the Empire State Games masters division later that summer placed second in the 50 meter freestyle, age 60–64, in a time of 36.43 seconds. In January, 2007 I was timed at 1:18.31 in the 100 yard freestyle.

My rising PSA has been kept under control by a regime of intermittent Casodex. An experimental treatment, it avoids the harsh side effects associated with a complete androgen blockage involving both Lupron injections and Casodex. The Casodex brings my PSA down to <0.1 ng/ml at which point I go off of it and my PSA rises again. When it rises to 8.0, I begin the

Casodex again. Eventually, my cancer will become resistant to the Casodex. I am presently in the third cycle of this treatment and at 11 years post-diagnosis am still without any symptoms or signs of metastasis.

Nothing has changed yet everything has changed. I continue to train and compete in sprints in spite of the cancer, my forte in swimming being identical to that as a runner. Beth has supported me and helped my psychological adjustment to the loss of running, a grieving not unlike the loss of a loved one. Since swimming had been a part of my cross-training as a runner, I was able to adjust readily to a new primary sport. Physically, my hip has healed nicely following surgery and my swimming is as strong now as it was prior to the accident. My philosophy of exercise and its benefits to men with prostate cancer has not changed and I continue to live out that philosophy. Having bought a new road bike to replace the one that crashed, I have now completed rides around five of the largest finger lakes, the longest a 78 mile jaunt around Seneca Lake.

References

AICR. 2002. What we know about diet and prostate cancer. American Institute for Cancer Research Newsletter 77:8–9.

Armstrong, L. 2001. It's Not About the Bike: My Journey Back To Life. Lance Armstrong with Sally Jenkins. The Berkeley Publishing Group, New York. 289p.

Aronowitz, J. 2002. Rational management of prostatectomy failure. Minutes of the October 25, 2001 meeting of the Syracuse Bob Dermody Chapter of the American Cancer Society's Man to Man Prostate Cancer Awareness and Support Group. Volume 9(4): 13–20.

Barnard, R. J., T. H. Ngo, P. Leung, W. J. Aronson and L. A. Golding. 2003. A low-fat diet and/or strenuous exercise alters the IGF axis in vivo and reduces prostate tumor cell growth in vitro. The Prostate 56: 201–206.

Booth, F. W. and P. D. Neufer. 2004. Exercise controls gene expression. American Scientist 93: 28–35.

Bortz, II, W. M. 1996. Dare to be 100: 99 steps to a long, healthy life. Fireside Book, Simon and Schuster, Inc., New York. 268p.

Bramble, D. M. and D. E. Lieberman. 2004. Endurance running and the evolution of Homo. Nature 432: 345–352.

Catalona, W. J. 2005. PSA tests are not all the same. Quest 14(3): 4–5.

Catalona, W. J. 2006. Dr. Catalona's response to DaVinci Robotics. Quest 15(2): 5.

Catalona, W. J., D. S. Smith, T. L. Ratliff, K. M. Dodds, D. E. Coplen, J. J. Yuan, J. A. Petros and G. L. Andriole. 1991. Measurement of prostate-specific antigen in a serum as a screening test for prostate cancer. New England Journal of Medicine 324(17): 1156–1161. Erratum in: New England Journal of Medicine 325(18): 1324; Comment in: New England Journal of Medicine 325: 963–965.

Catalona, W. J. and D. S. Smith. 1994. 5-year tumor recurrence rates after anatomical radical retropubic prostatectomy for prostate cancer. The Journal of Urology 152: 1837–1842.

Catalona, W. J. 2007. Being overweight can affect prostate cancer aggressiveness. Quest 16(1): 15.

Clingan, D. and L. Patz. 2004. Masters Track & Field Rankings (2003). National Masters News. March, 2004, pp 15–22.

Cooper, K. H. 1970. The New Aerobics. Bantam Press, New York. 191p.

Dorai, T., N. Gehani and A. Katz. 2000. "Therapeutic potential of Curcumin in human prostate cancer-l. Curcumin induces apoptosis in both androgen-dependent and androgen-independent prostate cancer cells." Prostate Cancer Prostatic Dis. 3(2): 84–93.

Eisenberg, L. 1996. Reality, humor and my prostate. New Choices, July/August, pp. 54–57.

Galik, K., B. Senut, M. Pickford, D. Gommery, J. Treil, A. J. Kuperavage and R. B. Eckhardt. 2004. External and internal morphology of the BAR 1002'00 Orrorin tugenensis femur. Science 305: 1450–1453.

Holden, C. (ed.) 2000. Six million-year-old man. In: Random Samples. Science 290:2065.

Jagetia, G. C. and B. B. Aggarwal. 2007. "Spicing up" of the immune system by curcumin. J. Clin. Immunol. 1: 19–35.

Kempermann, G., H. G. Kuhn and F. H. Gage. 1997. More hippocampus neurons in adult mice living in an enriched environment. Nature 386: 493–495.

Korda, M. 1996. Man to Man: Surviving Prostate Cancer. Random House, New York.

Lazarov, O., J. Robinson, Y.-P. Tang, L. S. Hairston, Z. Korade-Mirnics, V. M.-Y. Lee, L. B. Hersh, R. M. Sapolsky, K. Mirnics and S. S. Sisodia. 2005. Environmental enrichment reduces Aß levels and amyloid deposition in transgenic mice. Cell 120: 701–713.

Lee, K. W., H. J. Lee, K. Kang and C Y. Lee. 2002. Preventive effects of vitamin C on carcinogenesis. The Lancet 359:172.

Lee, S. H., T. Oe and I. A. Blair. 2001. Vitamin-C induced decomposition of lipid hydroperoxides to endogenous genotoxins. Science 292:2083–2086.

Lee, I.-M. and R. S. Paffenbarger, Jr. 2000. Associations of light, moderate, and vigorous intensity physical activity with longevity. The Harvard Alumni Health Study. Am. J. Epidemiology 151:293–299.

Letters to the Editor. 2001. Science's Compass. Science 293:1993–1995.

Levy, D. H. 1999. Advice from a patient who has been there. Parade Magazine, January 17, 1999, pp. 14–15.

Narla, G., K. E. Heath, H. L. Reeves, D. Li, L. E. Giono, A. C. Kimmelman, M. J. Glucksman, J. Narla, F. J. Eng, A. M. Chan, A. C. Ferrari, J. A. Martignetti and S. L. Friedman. 2001. KLF6, a candidate tumor suppressor gene mutated in prostate cancer. Science 294: 2563–2566.

Narla, G., A. DiFeo, H. L. Reeves, D. J. Schaid, J. Hirshfeld, E. Hod, A. Katz, W. B. Isaacs, S. Hebbring, A. Komiya, S. K. McDonnell, K. E. Wiley, S. J. Jacobsen, S. D. Isaacs, P. C. Walsh, S. L. Zheng, B.-L.

Chang, D. M. Friedrichsen, J. L. Stanford, E. A. Ostrander, A. M. Chinnaiyan, M. A. Rubin, J. Xu, S. N. Thibodeau, S. L. Friedman and J. A. Martignetti. 2005. A germline DNA polymorphism enhances alternative splicing of the KLF6 tumor suppressor gene and is associated with increased prostate cancer risk. Cancer Res. 65: 1213–1222.

National Cancer Institute. 2005. National Cancer Institute Fact Sheet. http://www.cancer.gov/cancertopics/factsheet/garlic-and-cancer-prevention.

Myers, Jr., C. E., S. S. Steck, and R. S. Myers. 2000. Eating Your Way to Better Health: The Prostate Forum Nutrition Guide. Rivanna Health Publications, Inc., Charlottesville, Virginia. 211p.

Pantuck, A. J., J. T. Leppert, N. Zomorodian, W. Aronson, J. Hong, R. J. Barnard, N. Seeram, H. Liker, H. Wang, R. Elashoff, D. Heber, M. Aviram, L. Ignarro and A. Belldegrun. 2006. Phase II study of pomegranate juice for men with rising prostate-specific antigen following surgery or radiation for prostate cancer. Clinical Cancer Research 12: 4018–4026.

Partin, A. W., W. J. Catalona, P. C. Southwick, E. N. Subong, G. H. Gasior and D. W. Chan. 1996. Analysis of percent free prostate-specific antigen (PSA) for prostate cancer detection: influence of total PSA, prostate volume, and age. Urology 48(6A Suppl): 55–61.

Pound, C. R., A. W. Partin, M. A. Eisenberger, D. W. Chan, J. D. Pearson and P. C. Walsh. 1999. The natural history of progression following PSA recurrence after radical prostatectomy. Journal of the American Medical Association 281: 1591–1597.

Pound, C. R., A. W. Partin, J. I. Epstein and P. C. Walsh. 1997. Prostate-specific antigen after anatomic radical retropubic prostatectomy. Patterns of recurrence and cancer control. Urologic Clinics of North America 24: 395–406.

Punglia, R. S., A. V. D'Amico, W. J. Catalona, K. A. Roehl and K. M. Kuntz. 2003. Effect of verification bias on screening for prostate cancer by measurement of prostate-specific antigen. New England Journal of Medicine 349: 335–342.

Rafii, S. and D. Lyden. 2005. VEGFR1-positive haematopoietic bone marrow progenitors initiate the pre-metastatic niche. Nature 438: 820–827.

Sesso, H. D., R. S. Paffenbarger, Jr., and I.-M. Lee. 2001. Alcohol consumption and risk of prostate cancer: The Harvard Alumni Health Study. Int. J. of Epidemiology 30: 749–755.

van Pragg, H., B. R. Christie, T. J. Sejnowski and F. H. Gage. 1999. Running enhances neurogenesis, learning, and long-term potentiation in mice. Proc. Natl. Acad. Sci. USA 96: 13427–13431.

van Pragg, H., A. F. Schinder, B. R. Christie, N. Toni, T. D. Palmer and F. H. Gage. 2002. Functional neurogenesis in the adult hippocampus. Nature 415: 1030–1034.

Walsh, P. C. 1995. The Prostate: A Guide for Men and the Women Who Love Them. Baltimore, MD; Johns Hopkins University Press.

Walsh, P. C. and J. F. Worthington. 2001. Dr. Patrick Walsh's Guide to Surviving Prostate Cancer. Warner Books, Inc., New York, New York. 462p.

Ward, J. F. and H. Zincke. 2003. Radical prostatectomy for the patient with locally advanced prostate cancer. Curr. Urol. Rep. 4(3): 196–204.

Ward, J. F., J. M. Slezak, M. L. Blute, E. J. Bergstralh and H. Zincke. 2005. Radical prostatectomy for clinically advanced (cT3) prostate cancer since the advent of prostate-specific antigen testing: 15-year outcome. BJU International 95: 751–756.

Zincke, H., J. E. Oersterling, M. L. Blute, E. J. Bergstralh, R. P. Myers and D. M. Barrett. 1994. Long-term (15 years) results after radical prostatectomy for clinically localized (stage T2c or lower) prostate cancer. The Journal of Urology 152: 1850–1857.

978-0-595-45830-1
0-595-45830-0